MEDICAL MANAGEMENT OF

PREGNANCY
Complicated
by DIABETES

FOURTH EDITION

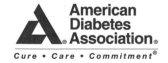

American
Diabetes
Association®

Cure • Care • Commitment®

Director, Book Publishing, Robert Anthony; *Managing Editor,* Abe Ogden; *Acquisitions, Professional Books,* Victor Van Beuren; *Editor,* Wendy Martin; *Production Manager,* Melissa Sprott; *Composition,* ADA; *Cover Design,* Koncept, Inc.; *Printer,* United Graphics Incorporated.

Printed in the United States of America
3 5 7 9 10 8 6 4

The suggestions and information contained in this publication are generally consistent with the *Clinical Practice Recommendations* and other policies of the American Diabetes Association, but they do not represent the policy or position of the Association or any of its boards or committees. Reasonable steps have been taken to ensure the accuracy of the information presented. However, the American Diabetes Association cannot ensure the safety or efficacy of any product or service described in this publication. Individuals are advised to consult a physician or other appropriate health care professional before undertaking any diet or exercise program or taking any medication referred to in this publication. Professionals must use and apply their own professional judgment, experience, and training and should not rely solely on the information contained in this publication before prescribing any diet, exercise, or medication. The American Diabetes Association—its officers, directors, employees, volunteers, and members—assumes no responsibility or liability for personal or other injury, loss, or damage that may result from the suggestions or information in this publication.

⊗ The paper in this publication meets the requirements of the ANSI Standard Z39.48-1992 (permanence of paper).

ADA titles may be purchased for business or promotional use or for special sales. To purchase more than 50 copies of this book at a discount, or for custom editions of this book with your logo, contact the American Diabetes Association at the address below, at booksales@diabetes.org, or by calling 703-299-2046.

American Diabetes Association
1701 North Beauregard Street
Alexandria, Virginia 22311

DOI: 10.2337/9781580402323

Library of Congress Cataloging-in-Publication Data

Medical management of pregnancy complicated by diabetes / [editor-in-chief], Lois B.
    Jovanovic. -- 4th ed.
        p. ; cm.
Includes bibliographical references and index.
ISBN 978-1-58040-232-3 (alk. paper)
1. Diabetes in pregnancy. I. Jovanovic, Lois B. II. American Diabetes Association.
[DNLM: 1. Pregnancy in Diabetics--therapy. WQ 248 M489 2009]
RG580.D5M43 2009
618.3--dc22
                                2008053962

Contents

A Word About This Guide

Pregnancy complicated by preexisting diabetes, be it type 1 or type 2 diabetes, is an example of a problem that can be minimized with a program of intensive and expert protocols and patient partnership to achieve the goals. There is no such thing as easy diabetes that can be treated as a secondary issue. Even mild, diet-controlled type 2 diabetes needs special attention to assure the mother of a normal, healthy infant. It is almost as if the more energy input by the health care team into the education and treatment of a diabetic pregnant woman, the better the outcome. The patient cannot be expected to sustain the motivation of an intensive care program without the sustained interaction of the health care team.

Gestational diabetes can also be addressed with intensive care programs, but this disease requires that additional energy be placed on the process of screening and diagnosis of the disease before the signs and symptoms are detected in the mother and fetus. Once the diagnosis is made, meticulous attention must be directed toward achieving and maintaining normoglycemia.

This book is intended to present to the clinician a complete package of protocols that have resulted in healthy infants in pregnancies complicated by type 1, type 2, or gestational diabetes.

Our first edition essentially followed these recommendations in that we emphasized individual meal plans to achieve normoglycemia under the instruction of a registered dietitian. The second edition incorporated the American Diabetes Association's 1994 Nutrition Recommendations and Principles for People with Diabetes Mellitus. In the third edition, we incorporated the nutrition recommendations for medical nutrition therapy and tailored them for the pregnant diabetic woman. This fourth edition contains the new guidelines for treatment with new insulin analogs, a discussion about the use of oral hypoglycemic agents in pregnancy, and the latest in obstetrical surveillance of the pregnant woman with diabetes.

Each contributor to this book has acknowledged that there are many ways to achieve the same excellent outcome, but each has also presented his or her preferred way to achieve the desired outcome. References to other protocols or a bibliography are given at the end of each section. You are invited to read the referenced protocols and come to your own conclusions, but it should be clear that a healthy pregnancy is only possible when each member of the health care team puts in the requisite extra attention and effort. After reading this book, it should be clear to every member of the team how much extra attention is required.

LOIS JOVANOVIČ, MD
Editor-in-Chief

Contributors

EDITOR-IN-CHIEF
Lois Jovanovič, MD
CEO and Chief Scientific Officer
Sansum Diabetes Research Institute

Clinical Professor of Medicine
University of Southern California
Keck School of Medicine

Adjunct Professor, Biomolecular
    Science and Engineering
University of California
Santa Barbara, California

Acknowledgments

The Editor gratefully acknowledges the contributions of the following health care professionals to this new edition:

Anne M. Patterson, RD, MPH
Director, WIC Program,
    Santa Barbara County
Director, Nutrition Programs,
    Santa Barbara County Health
    Department

Lisa Marasco, MA, IBCLC, FILCA
Lactation Consultant,
Private Practice and Santa Barbara
    County Public Health Department
    Nutrition Services/WIC
    Santa Maria, CA

Sue Kirkman, MD
Vice President, Clinical Affairs,
    American Diabetes Association

Stephanie Dunbar, MPH, RD
Director, Clinical Affairs,
    American Diabetes Association

We would also like to acknowledge the contributions of the following health care professionals and members of the Association's Professional Section to previous editions of this work:

John L. Kitzmiller, MD
Santa Clara Valley Medical Center
Department of Obstetrics
San Jose, California

Donald R. Coustan, MD
Department of Obstetrics and
    Gynecology
Brown University School of Medicine
and Women and Infants' Hospital of
    Rhode Island
Providence, Rhode Island

Richard M. Cowett, MD
Department of Pediatrics
Brown University School of Medicine
and Women and Infants' Hospital of
    Rhode Island
Providence, Rhode Island

Donna Jornsay, RN, BSN, CPNP, CDE
Division of Maternal Fetal Medicine
North Shore University Hospital
Manhasset, New York

Noreen Hall Papatheodorou, MSS,
    ACSW
Universal Health Associates, Inc.
Washington, DC

Prepregnancy Counseling and Management of Women with Preexisting Diabetes or Previous Gestational Diabetes

Highlights
Prepregnancy Counseling and Management of Women with Preexisting Diabetes or Previous Gestational Diabetes

■ With proper counseling and management by the primary care physician, the outcome of most pregnancies complicated by diabetes can approach that for the general population.

■ General guidelines for prepregnancy counseling and management of women with preexisting diabetes are:

- Ensure that pregnancy is planned; counsel the woman about contraception methods.
- Clearly identify for the woman and her partner the risks of congenital anomalies and spontaneous abortions and their relation to glucose control.
- Provide realistic information about chronic complications of type 1 diabetes, their potential impact on pregnancy and childbearing, and the effect of pregnancy on chronic complications.
- Assess the woman's fitness for pregnancy, paying special attention to retinopathy, nephropathy, hypertension, neuropathy, and ischemic heart disease.
- Identify any gynecologic abnormalities before conception, and treat infertility as early as possible in view of the risk to pregnancy associated with increasing duration of diabetes and advancing maternal age. Social, financial, and marital

factors permitting, pregnancy should be encouraged.

- Provide genetic counseling, including the risks of advanced maternal age, if applicable.
- Provide realistic information about additional medical costs associated with a pregnancy complicated by diabetes, such as extra office visits, possible hospitalization, special tests, and possible intensive neonatal care.
- Achieve optimum control of blood glucose levels before conception. Ideally, A1C should be normal or near normal before discontinuing contraception.
- Encourage good general principles of health, nutrition, and hygiene, including cessation of smoking and alcohol consumption. Prescribe a prenatal vitamin with folate as part of the preconception treatment plan.
- Identify any problems requiring psychosocial consultation.
- Once the decision is made to attempt pregnancy, provide appropriate optimism that careful glycemic control and meticulous obstetric care results in an excellent outcome in the vast majority of patients.
- Diagnose pregnancy as early as

possible and document conception date.

■ **Counseling and management of women with previous gestational diabetes should include:**
- Measuring glucose levels and assessing the need for further glucose tolerance testing or treatment if diabetes or impaired glucose tolerance is found.
- Evaluating weight status and advising weight reduction if appropriate.
- Reviewing risks:
  – Gestational diabetes in future pregnancy (~60–70% risk).
  – Type 2 diabetes (~50–75% risk if woman is obese).

- Advising careful family planning with use of effective contraceptive until pregnancy is desired.

■ **Problems remaining in the care of pregnant women with diabetes are:**
- Higher incidence of congenital anomalies and spontaneous abortions than in the nondiabetic population.
- The woman with severe complications of diabetes.
- The "difficult" or nonadherent patient.
- Education of caregivers and women with diabetes during childbearing years regarding the importance of preconception planning and care.

Prepregnancy Counseling and Management of Women with Preexisting Diabetes or Previous Gestational Diabetes

Women with diabetes in pregnancy are divided into two categories: *1)* those with diabetes that predates the pregnancy and *2)* those whose diabetes develops during the pregnancy, known as gestational diabetes mellitus (GDM). In both categories, when left untreated, the diabetes can significantly increase the risk of maternal and fetal/neonatal morbidity and mortality. Prepregnancy care incorporated into the plan of management for women with preexisting diabetes can result in improved pregnancy outcomes. This chapter provides the rationale behind and protocols for developing a prepregnancy program for women with diabetes or who have had previous gestational diabetes.

PREEXISTING DIABETES

Women with preexisting diabetes (type 1 or type 2) who desire pregnancy present a broad array of challenging problems for the primary care physician and obstetrician. In the preinsulin era, maternal mortality was as high as 44%, and perinatal mortality was 60% (1). However, true type 1 diabetic children did not live to childbearing ages. After the discovery of insulin, maternal and fetal/neonatal survival improved dramatically. During the past three decades, advances in the care of the individual with diabetes in general, as well as advances in fetal surveillance and neonatal care, have continued to improve outcomes in most diabetic pregnancies to near that of the general population (2,3). The most common maternal (Table 1) and fetal/neonatal (Table 2) complications have been decreased dramatically.

Despite the advances made in the care of the pregnant woman with diabetes, several problems remain:

- A high prevalence of congenital anomalies and spontaneous abortions (SABs) in infants of diabetic mothers (IDMs)
- Care of the woman with severe complications of diabetes
- Care of the "difficult patient" who often presents late for antenatal care and/or is nonadherent (4)

Morbidity and mortality associated with major congenital anomalies and SAB are of major concern. The magnitude of both appears to be related to metabolic control. The true prevalence of SAB in diabetic pregnancies is not known but has been reported to be as high as 30–60%, depending on the degree of hyperglycemia at the time of conception, double that of the general population (5). The increased risk of congenital anomalies in IDMs ranges from 6 to 12%, a two- to fivefold

Table 1 Maternal Complications in Diabetic Pregnancy

- Hypoglycemia, ketoacidosis
- Pregnancy-induced hypertension
- Pyelonephritis, other infections
- Polyhydramnios
- Preterm labor
- Worsening of chronic complications—retinopathy, nephropathy, neuropathy, cardiac disease

increase over the 2–3% incidence observed in the general population (6,7). This increased risk of congenital anomalies accounts for ~40% of the perinatal loss in IDMs (8). The combined risk of congenital anomalies and SAB in poorly controlled diabetes in early pregnancy can approach 65% (9).

The types of congenital anomalies observed in infants of diabetic mothers (IDMs) are varied (Table 3). Most are of cardiac, neural tube, or skeletal origin; they are more commonly multiple, more severe, and more often fatal than those found in the general population.

The etiology of this increased prevalence of congenital anomalies in IDMs has been the subject of intense research in recent years. In an experimental setting, hyperglycemia and other metabolic abnormalities are teratogenic, singly or in combination (8–12). Fetal organogenesis is largely complete by 8 wk after the last menstrual period (6 wk postconception) (13). Poorly controlled diabetes during the early weeks of pregnancy, in many cases before a woman even knows that she has conceived, significantly increases the risk of a first-trimester SAB or delivering an infant with a major anomaly (14).

The A1C, which expresses an average of the circulating glucose for the 4–6 wk before its measurement, has become a useful tool in assessing a woman's metabolic control early in pregnancy, during the critical period of organogenesis. Several studies have shown a definite association between A1C levels in early pregnancy (<13 wk) and increased risk of congenital anomalies and SABs (14–16; Fig. 1).

Table 2 Potential Perinatal Morbidity/Mortality in Infants of Diabetic Mothers

■ Asphyxia	■ Increased red blood cells
■ Birth injury	■ Intrauterine growth retardation
■ Cardiac hypertrophy	■ Macrosomia
■ Congenital anomalies	■ Neurological instability; irritability
■ Erythremia and hyperviscosity	■ Organomegaly
■ Heart failure	■ Respiratory distress
■ Hyperbilirubinemia	■ Respiratory distress syndrome
■ Hypocalcemia	■ Small left colon syndrome
■ Hypoglycemia	■ Stillbirth
■ Hypomagnesemia	■ Transient hematuria

Table 3 Congenital Malformations in Infants of Diabetic Mothers

Anomaly	Ratios of Incidence
Caudal regression	252
Spina bifida, hydrocephalus, or other CNS defect	2
Anencephalus	3
Heart anomalies	4
Anal/rectal atresia	3
Renal anomalies	5
Agenesis	6
Cystic kidney	4
Ureter duplex	23
Situs inversus	84

Ratio of incidence is in comparison to the general population. Adapted from Mills et al. (13). Heart anomalies include transposition of the great vessels, ventricular septal defect, and atrial septal defect.

As a result of these findings, high-risk perinatal centers have developed programs for preconceptional management of the diabetic woman planning a pregnancy. Women in these centers are evaluated and counseled about the risks of pregnancy, with particular emphasis on the importance of normalizing blood glucose levels periconceptionally to reduce the risks of delivering an infant with a major birth defect. Studies from these centers have confirmed that normalizing blood glucose levels before and during the early weeks of pregnancy can reduce the risk of development of major anomalies, as well as the occurrence of SAB in IDMs, to near that of the nondiabetic population (14,17–19).

Thus, prepregnancy counseling and management have emerged as vital components in the care of the woman with diabetes (20). The goals of such a program are listed in Table 4. A practical method for organizing and implementing a program for preconceptional care is outlined in this chapter. Major topics include prepregnancy counseling, assessment, and management.

PREPREGNANCY COUNSELING

Prepregnancy counseling for the woman with diabetes ideally should begin at the onset of puberty and continue until permanent sterilization or menopause, thus encompassing all women with diabetes of childbearing potential. Furthermore, these women should be divided into two categories—those planning a pregnancy within the next year and those wanting to delay pregnancy. For women not planning a pregnancy in the near future, general information can be given regarding the risks of pregnancy and the importance of appropriate birth control and prepregnancy planning. Even the teenage girl who may not be thinking in terms of pregnancy needs to be questioned regarding her menstrual history and sexual activity. Her physician should provide her with information about the importance of planning one's family in the future.

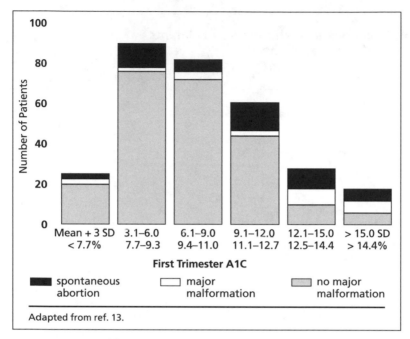

Figure 1. Major malformations and spontaneous abortions according to 1st-trimester A1C.

For the woman contemplating pregnancy soon, a preconception consultation with her physician is essential. The major components of preconception counseling include:

- Contraceptive advice
- Risks of pregnancy, maternal and fetal/neonatal
- Importance of maintaining normal blood glucose levels
- Genetic counseling
- Personal commitment by the woman and her family

A planned pregnancy is a major objective of preconception counseling; thus, establishing an effective contraceptive method must be an early priority in prepregnancy planning (see also page 28). The physician should review with the woman her options for contraception and help her choose the one most appropriate for her situation.

The physician should next explain to the woman the risks of pregnancy to her developing baby as well as to herself (Table 1; see also page 140). This prepregnancy counseling session is the ideal moment to emphasize to the woman her two- to fivefold increased risk of having a baby with a congenital anomaly and her increased risk for having a first-trimester SAB. This is the crucial time to underscore these particular problems so that the patient will understand fully the ratio-

Table 4 Goals of Prepregnancy Planning Program

- Assessment of a woman's fitness for pregnancy
- Obstetric evaluation
- Intensive education of woman and family
- Attainment of optimum diabetic control
- Timing and planning of pregnancy

nale behind preconception care with the effort toward normalizing blood glucose levels before and during the early weeks of pregnancy. She should be apprised that organogenesis is largely complete by the eighth week of gestation after her last menstrual period and that, with efforts to normalize blood glucose levels, her risk for having a baby with a congenital anomaly or an early SAB can be reduced significantly (Fig. 1). Furthermore, she can be assured that with continued optimal glucose control throughout pregnancy, she can effectively reduce her risk of developing further complications.

Next, the physician should advise the woman of her own personal risks when undertaking pregnancy, emphasizing to her the need for evaluation for the presence of diabetic complications and other general medical problems before conception. She will need to know that the chronic complications of diabetes can worsen during pregnancy, although debate still remains as to whether the pregnancy itself influences the natural course of these complications. Certainly, retinopathy has been known to progress in some patients during pregnancy (21–35). If the woman has known renal insufficiency or severe gastroenteropathy, she should be advised that these conditions constitute significant risks to both mother and developing infant and may be, in some individuals, contraindications to pregnancy. The presence of ischemic heart disease, known to be associated with significant maternal mortality, is in most cases a contraindication to pregnancy. Thus, preconception evaluation of these potential complications must be emphasized.

Although these risks are obviously serious, emphasis can be placed on the evidence accumulated to date—namely, that for most women, intensive management of the diabetes with the goal of normalizing blood glucose levels before and during the entire pregnancy can result in outcomes similar to those of the non-diabetic population (36).

Genetics is another important aspect of preconception counseling. The woman with diabetes may be reassured that it is rare for a newborn to develop diabetes. If she has type 1 diabetes and is ≥25 yr old, the chance of her child developing diabetes at some point is ~1%; if she is <25 yr old, this chance increases to ~4% (37). If both parents have type 1 diabetes, the risk is not known but is expected to be somewhat higher, but still less than 10%. The risk for offspring of women with type 2 diabetes to eventually develop type 2 diabetes is about double the risk of the general population (37). Although these risks of developing diabetes are higher than that of the general population, they are not significant enough to advise a woman against pregnancy on genetic grounds.

Finally, the physician must convey to each woman the importance of the deep personal commitment that she will be undertaking during the pregnancy. The demands of maintaining a routine to normalize the blood glucose are many. For some patients, the actual cost of such an undertaking may be prohibitive. The woman needs to understand that once pregnant, she will be seen frequently by her primary care physician or endocrinologist as well as her obstetrician, perhaps as often as weekly. She may require hospitalization if problems with the pregnancy develop or her metabolic control deteriorates. She will be undergoing various special tests throughout the pregnancy to assess the well-being of her developing baby. She may want to check with her insurance company to see what coverage her policy offers with regard to pregnancy. Many states offer supplemental aid programs to indigent women during pregnancy. The patient can seek help through her local health department or her state's maternal/child health division.

In addition, the physician may also want to have the woman undergo psychosocial evaluation and counseling. The counselor can assist her in coping with the specific problems pertaining to pregnancy and other pressing commitments such as small children in the family, job responsibilities, and financial burdens. If, after discussing in depth these various aspects of diabetes and pregnancy and the commitment required, the woman decides that she would like to pursue a pregnancy, she can then be scheduled for prepregnancy assessment.

PREPREGNANCY ASSESSMENT

The prepregnancy assessment of a woman with diabetes (Table 5) should begin with a detailed diabetic history, including:

- Type of diabetes
- Age of onset, duration, and course of disease
- Past history, including hospitalizations for treatment of acute and chronic complications
- Current diabetic regimen, with attention to routine insulin dosages, prior or current use of oral glucose-lowering agents, medical nutrition therapy and individualized meal plan, exercise, hypoglycemia unawareness, and self-monitoring of blood glucose
- History of other medical problems, especially hypertension and thyroid disease

Table 5 Prepregnancy Assessment for Diabetic Women

■History and physical examination
■Gynecologic evaluation
■Laboratory evaluation
- A1C level
- Urinalysis and culture
- 24-h urine for creatinine clearance and total protein
- Thyroid panel: free T4 1.0–1.6 and TSH <2.5 µU/l
■Special studies
- Electrocardiogram or treadmill
- Neuropathy testing if indicated

- A careful obstetric history with attention to contraceptive use and past history of infertility or pregnancy complications such as pregnancy-induced hypertension, polyhydramnios, and preterm labor
- All medications that the patient is taking
- A support system, including family and work environment

The physician should then perform a careful physical examination with special attention not only to diabetes-related complications, but also to other organ-system abnormalities not directly related to diabetes, especially hypertension. Known hypertension in a woman with diabetes should be treated promptly with medications not known to be teratogenic, such as methyldopa and hydralozine. Angiotensin-converting enzyme (ACE) inhibitors are contraindicated in pregnancy because of their association with neonatal renal failure and pregnancy loss.

The following are recommendations concerning blood pressure control in pregnancy (38–50):

- Nonpregnant diabetic patients with hypertension should be treated to a blood pressure <130 mmHg systolic and <80 mmHg diastolic.
- In the possible interest of long-term maternal health, we recommend blood pressure treatment targets of 110–129 mmHg systolic and 65–79 mmHg diastolic for diabetic pregnant women with chronic hypertension until there is clear evidence from randomized clinical trials that the fetal risk from treatment of hypertension exceeds maternal benefit. Too tight control of maternal blood pressure may limit fetal growth or cause limb defects.
- Pregnant diabetic patients with chronic hypertension should receive drug therapy in addition to lifestyle and behavioral therapy. In mid-pregnancy, drug dosage may need to be reduced.
- Drugs safe for pregnancy should be added sequentially until target blood pressure levels are achieved.
- ACE inhibitors and angiotensin receptor blockers are contraindicated in pregnancy.
- Atenolol may be associated with a greater risk of small-for-gestational-age infants and should be avoided.
- Patients not achieving target blood pressure despite multiple drug therapy should be referred to a physician experienced in the care of pregnant diabetic patients with hypertension.
- All diabetic women, especially those with hypertension, should be closely monitored for the development of preeclampsia.
- Twenty-four–hour ambulatory blood pressure monitoring or blood pressure self-measurements may provide a more complete picture of the blood pressure burden than isolated office blood pressure and should be considered when determining the need for or monitoring the effect of antihypertensive therapy.

The woman's eye examination must be performed through dilated pupils by an ophthalmologist. If this examination reveals preproliferative retinopathy or macular edema, proper treatment, including laser photocoagulation, should be performed and the woman's retinal status stabilized before pregnancy. Risk factors for progression of retinopathy include:

- Duration of diabetes
- Retinal status
- Elevated A1C
- Hypertension
- Valsalva maneuver (increases risk of retinal hemorrhage)

Likewise, a careful evaluation of the patient's renal status and efforts to detect the presence of autonomic and peripheral neuropathies are important.

The possible presence of cardiac disease must be evaluated carefully. If a woman has had diabetes for >10 yr, or any duration of diabetes and hypertension, the physician should consider obtaining an electrocardiogram and perhaps even proceed with more in-depth cardiac testing to rule out underlying ischemic heart disease, especially if the woman gives a history of chest pain.

The woman should also have a neurological assessment and lower-extremity examination for evidence of vascular disease, neuropathy, deformity, or infection (34).

In addition to this thorough medical assessment, the woman should undergo a careful gynecologic examination. Prompt detection and treatment of gynecologic abnormalities such as infection or structural deformities are advantageous. Additionally, it is important to determine whether the woman has any degree of infertility, so that a specific problem can be treated early to minimize any delay for the planned pregnancy.

Finally, as part of the woman's total evaluation, the physician should order the following specific baseline laboratory studies in addition to those relating to the woman's general medical status:

- Initial A1C level to evaluate her current degree of metabolic control
- Renal function, including a 24-h urine collection for creatinine clearance and total protein and microalbumin
- Clean-catch urinalysis with culture and sensitivity
- Thyroid testing that would include free T4, thyroid-stimulating hormone (TSH) level, and anti-microsomal antibodies (39)

On completion of the preconception assessment, the patient will see her physician for a return counseling appointment. At that visit, her physician will review with her the results of her tests and discuss her fitness for pregnancy.

Table 6 Potential Contraindications to Pregnancy

- Ischemic heart disease
- Active proliferative retinopathy, untreated
- Renal insufficiency: creatinine clearance <50 ml/min or serum creatinine >2 mg/dl or heavy proteinuria (>2 g/24 h) or hypertension (blood pressure >130/80 mmHg despite treatment)
- Severe gastroenteropathy: nausea/vomiting, diarrhea

The discovery of certain diabetes-related complications may serve as absolute or relative contraindications for pregnancy (Table 6). If the woman is found to have clinically proven cardiac disease, the risks of maternal mortality are high, and the woman with this very serious complication should be counseled against undertaking pregnancy. Additionally, she should be asked to consider permanent sterilization.

If the woman is found to have significant proliferative retinopathy, she should be advised to delay the pregnancy until the ophthalmologist can treat her eye disease appropriately and determine that the retinopathy has stabilized.

If she displays significant renal disease (serum creatinine >2 mg/dl and/or creatinine clearance <50 ml/min), she must be warned about the high risk of morbidity and mortality of her infant that is associated with this particular complication. Likewise, significant proteinuria (>300 mg/24 h), especially when accompanied by hypertension, portends a poor pregnancy outcome (1). Proteinuria >2 g/24 h is a potential contraindication to pregnancy.

Women with nephropathy are at increased risk to develop hypertension and significant edema to the extent that it interrupts their lifestyle. A woman who has undergone renal transplantation may be able to undertake pregnancy safely if her medical status is otherwise stable, although the risk is still significant.

Severe gastroenteropathy should be considered a relative contraindication to pregnancy. Metabolic control and nutrition for both the woman and her developing baby are difficult to maintain with this particular complication.

In conclusion, if the woman shows no evidence of active diabetic complications or other health problems that place her at significant risk, she may be safely advised to begin plans for pregnancy. At this point, she may be entered into the prepregnancy management protocol.

PREPREGNANCY MANAGEMENT

Once a woman has undergone prepregnancy counseling and assessment and her fitness for safely undertaking a pregnancy has been established, her physician should outline a plan for prepregnancy management, the goal of which is to normalize the blood glucose levels before conception and to maintain euglycemia throughout the pregnancy.

Assuming that all preexisting complications of a woman's diabetes have been stabilized, she can then be introduced to the team concept of patient management. Ideally, her diabetes team should include:

- Her primary care physician and endocrinologist
- Her obstetrician, who is skilled in high-risk obstetrics
- A nurse educator (preferably a certified diabetes educator)
- A social worker
- A registered dietitian
- A pediatrician or neonatologist

She should undergo individual consultations with both the nurse educator and dietitian, who will assess her current routine and level of knowledge concerning her diabetes. Her caloric needs based on height, weight, age, and activity level can be calculated and a meal plan developed with a calorie content that will

Table 7 Prepregnancy Diet Calculation

■ Determination of daily calorie requirement:
  • 30–34 kcal/kg (2.2 lb) pre-gravid body weight for normal-weight woman (BMI <25)
  • 23–25 kcal/kg (2.2 lb) pre-gravid body weight for obese woman (BMI ≥30)
  • To lose 1 lb/wk, subtract 500 kcal from daily requirement or increase exercise
■ Distribution of calories:
  • Variable carbohydrate (consistent amount of daily carbohydrate intake may be beneficial)
  • Saturated fat intake <7% of total calories
  • Intake of trans fat minimized
  • Dietary cholesterol limited to <200 mg/day

help her attain or maintain her ideal body weight and glycemic control (40) (Table 7). Folate given periconceptually and in early pregnancy decreases the risk of neural tube defects in offspring. Therefore, prescribing a prenatal vitamin containing a minimum of 400 mg folate from preconception and throughout is recommended.

Next, the woman should be placed on an intensive regimen of multiple injections in a basal-bolus fashion (Tables 8 and 9), or an insulin pump if she is not already practicing an intensive regimen. If the woman has been treated with oral hypoglycemic agents, these must be discontinued and insulin therapy initiated.

Insulin is the mainstay of therapy for preexisting diabetes in pregnancy. Intensive insulin therapy with either three or four injections of insulin/day or the use of an insulin pump is necessary in most patients to achieve the near-normal blood glucose goals that are defined above. Both multiple daily injections (MDIs) and continuous subcutaneous insulin infusion (CSII) use the concept of basal and bolus insulin replacement in an attempt to mimic normal physiologic delivery of insulin during fasting and eating. Skills for intensive diabetes self-management are best learned before pregnancy, so that excellent glycemic control is achieved at the time of conception and during organogenesis. Unfortunately, this is not always possible, since many women have unplanned pregnancies and have suboptimal self-management skills. However, a woman's strong motivation to care for her fetus by improving her diabetes control offers a window of opportunity to teach her skills that she may continue to use for the rest of her life.

Basal insulin is used to approximate the fasting insulin requirements. When MDI therapy is used, intermediate-acting insulins such as NPH are used two to three times per day to provide basal coverage. NPH peaks at 4 h and has a duration of action of ~13 h. Daytime and nighttime hypoglycemia is common in diabetic pregnancies (51,52). The relatively short peak action profile of NPH may explain the high risk of nocturnal hypoglycemia, even when taken at bedtime, in the setting of the low fasting glucose treatment goals established for pregnancy. A bedtime snack is usually needed to reduce this risk. Middle-of-the-night blood glucose levels should be spot-checked once or twice a month or more often depending on the clinical situation. The morning dose of intermediate-acting insulin should be given within 8–10 h after the bedtime dose to

Table 8 Sample Prepregnancy Daily Insulin Therapy

■ **Goals of therapy**
- Fasting, premeal blood glucose 70–100 mg/dl
- 1-h postmeal blood glucose <120 mg/dl (<6.7 mmol/l)
- A1C at or near upper limit of normal range: for example, if normal range is 4.7–6.1%, A1C should be <6.1%

avoid hyperglycemia as the nighttime insulin concentration is waning. Pre-dinner dosing of intermediate-acting insulin should be avoided, since the risks of nocturnal hypoglycemia and fasting hyperglycemia are increased. A lunchtime injection of intermediate-acting insulin may be needed to prevent pre-dinner hyperglycemia.

The long-acting insulin analog glargine provides steady serum levels over 24 h in patients who are not pregnant, but concerns related to its increased binding to the insulin-like growth factor (IGF) receptor and lack of safety data in pregnancy exclude it from use in pregnancy at this time (see below). The long-acting analog detemir is also not recommended. CSII uses a short- or rapid-acting insulin delivered by continuous infusion to deliver a small predetermined amount of insulin per hour. Steady-state basal levels of insulin are achieved. Titration of the basal insulin dose is based on the premeal glucose value, since serial fasting is not done during pregnancy.

Bolus insulin treatment requires an understanding of medical nutrition therapy. Short- or rapid-acting insulin is given when carbohydrate is ingested. Short- or rapid-acting insulin may be given with a set meal plan that involves consistent carbohydrate at meals and snacks or based on a predetermined insulin-to-carbohydrate ratio allowing for more flexible carbohydrate intake. A correction dose based on an empiric or calculated sensitivity factor is given to treat an elevated glucose value. Titration of the bolus insulin level is based on the trends of the postprandial glucose value. This approach to bolus insulin is used with both MDI and CSII.

MDI and CSII each have advantages and disadvantages. CSII offers multiple programmable basal rates that can be especially useful for patients with nocturnal hypoglycemia and a prominent dawn phenomenon. The disadvantage of CSII is the potential for marked hyperglycemia and diabetic ketoacidosis as a consequence of insulin delivery failure. This can occur when technical problems arise with the pump or more often when there is kinking of the catheter or when an air bubble in the tubing displaces insulin. Women who use CSII in pregnancy can take steps to avoid the serious problem of diabetic ketoacidosis by testing blood glucose levels before and after meals, at bedtime, and within 2 h of changing the infusion set. Patients should always test blood glucose levels and ketones if symptoms of hyperglycemia and especially nausea develop, although these symptoms can be masked by pregnancy symptoms. Blood glucose levels >180 mg/dl in the absence of urine ketones should be rechecked within 2 h of a high bolus to insure that glucose levels are improving. Glucose levels >180 mg/dl in the presence of urine ketones should be treated immediately with a subcutaneous injection. Blood

Table 9 Insulin Dosage Regimen for Diabetic Pregnancy

Pregnancy NPH plus rapid-acting insulin schedule

Patient weight in kg = _____ Date and time: _____

Big I = total daily units of insulin

Circle one: Gestational weeks =	0–12	13–28	29–34	35–40	OTHER
k =	0.7	0.8	0.9	1.0	

Calculate desired units of insulin from above line.
  Big I = _____ (k units × weight kg)/24 h
  Big I = Basal insulin requirement + Bolus (meal-related) insulin requirement
  Basal = ½ Big I, Bolus = ½ Big I
  Basal: Divide so that 1/6 of Big I is NPH given before breakfast, 1/6 of Big I is
      NPH given before dinner, and 1/6 of Big I is NPH given before bedtime.
  Bolus: Divide so that 1/6 of Big I is rapid-acting insulin given before breakfast,
      1/6 of Big I is rapid-acting insulin given before lunch, and 1/6 of Big I is
      rapid-acting insulin given before dinner. The rapid-acting insulin is then
      titrated based on the blood glucose.

0800 Pre-breakfast: NPH = 1/6 Big I = _____.
  Check yesterday's pre-dinner blood glucose (BG):
      If yesterday's pre-dinner BG <60, then decrease today's morning NPH by 2 U.
      If yesterday's pre-dinner BG 61–90, no change in today's morning NPH.
      If yesterday's pre-dinner BG >91, then increase today's morning NPH by 2 U.

Rapid-acting insulin = 1/6 Big I = _____ to be adjusted according to the
following scale:
      Pre-breakfast BG <60 = _____ = (1/6 Big I dose) − 3% of the Big I
      61–90   =   _____ = 1/6 Big I dose
      91–120 =   _____ = (1/6 Big I dose) + 3% of the Big I
      >121   =   _____ = (1/6 Big I dose) + 6% of the Big I

If today's BG 1 h after breakfast is <110, then decrease tomorrow's pre-breakfast
    rapid insulin by 2 U.
If today's BG 1 h after breakfast is 111–120, no change in tomorrow's pre-breakfast
    rapid insulin.
If today's BG 1 h after breakfast is >121, then increase tomorrow's pre-breakfast
    rapid insulin by 2 U.

---

glucose levels and urine ketones should be checked hourly. The infusion setup should be changed and glucose levels carefully reevaluated.

Five insulin analogs are approved by the Food and Drug Administration (FDA) for use in nonpregnant patients. The rapid-acting insulins may improve patient adherence, decrease postmeal glucose excursions, and lower the risk of nocturnal hypoglycemia. Of the three rapid-acting insulins, lispro, glulisinie, and aspart, lispro has been widely used in pregnancy without apparent adverse affects (51–69). Although large prospective randomized controlled clinical trials are not available, several retrospective and small prospective clinical trials support the safe use of lispro in pregnancy (51–69). Lispro does not appear to cross the pla-

1200 Pre-lunch: Rapid-acting insulin is 1/6 Big I = _____ to be adjusted according to the following scale:
       Pre-lunch BG <60 = _____ = (1/6 Big I dose) – 3% of Big I
       61–90 = _____ = 1/6 Big I dose
       91–120 = _____ = (1/6 Big I dose) + 3% of the Big I
       >121   = _____ = (1/6 Big I dose) + 6% of the Big I

If today's BG 1 h after lunch is <110, then decrease tomorrow's pre-lunch rapid insulin by 2 U.
If today's BG 1 h after lunch is 111–120, no change in tomorrow's pre-lunch rapid insulin.
If today's BG 1 h after lunch is >121, then increase tomorrow's pre-lunch rapid insulin by 2 U.

1700 Pre-dinner: NPH = 1/6 Big I = _____.
Rapid-acting insulin is 1/6 Big I = _____ to be adjusted according to the following scale:
    If yesterday's pre-bedtime BG is <60, then decrease today's dinner NPH by 2 U.
    If yesterday's pre-bedtime BG is 61–90, no change in today's dinner NPH.
    If yesterday's pre-bedtime BG is >91, then increase today's dinner NPH by 2 U.
       Pre-dinner BG <60 = _____ = (1/6 Big I dose) – 3% of Big I
       61–90 = _____ = 1/6 Big I dose
       91–120 = _____ = (1/6 Big I dose) + 3% of the Big I
       >121   = _____ = (1/6 Big I dose) + 6% of the Big I
If today's BG 1 h after dinner is <110, then decrease tomorrow's dinner rapid insulin by 2 U.
If today's BG 1 h after dinner is 111–120, no change in tomorrow's dinner rapid insulin.
If today's BG 1 h after dinner is >121, then increase tomorrow's dinner rapid insulin by 2 U.

2400 Bedtime NPH: Give 1/6 Big I = _____.
If today's pre-breakfast BG is <60, then decrease today's bedtime NPH by 2 U.
If today's pre-breakfast BG is 61–90, no change in today's bedtime NPH.
If today's pre-breakfast BG is >91, then check the 3 a.m. BG and, if it is <70 (regardless of today's pre-breakfast BG), decrease today's bedtime NPH by 2 U.
If today's pre-breakfast BG is >91 and the 3 a.m. BG is >70, increase today's bedtime NPH by 2 U.
Also, if the 3 a.m. BG is >91, then call the doctor for a 3 a.m. rapid insulin scale equal to the pre-lunch rapid scale.

---

centa. It does not appear to cause an increased incidence of congenital malformations, and it does not appear to cause an increased risk of progression of retinopathy. Both lispro and aspart appear to achieve lower 1- to 2-h postprandial glucoses levels in either gestational or preexisting diabetes compared with regular insulin (51–69). The FDA lists both lispro and aspart as safety category B. Data regarding the use of glargine in pregnancy are limited to case reports. Glargine is associated with a six- to eightfold increase in binding to the IGF receptor and mitogenic potency respectively compared with regular insulin (70,71). However, the mitogenic response of insulin relative to IGF-1 is ~1%. Thus, at physiologic concentrations, glargine may not display significant augmentation of mitogenic effects compared with regular insulin (70–72). The clinical significance of these binding and mitogenic effects is not known. Until more information is available, glargine should be avoided in pregnancy under most circumstances. Glargine is listed as category C by the FDA. There are no data on glulisine or detemir use in pregnancy, thus these insulins are also listed as category C.

Additionally, instruction in an appropriate exercise routine will enhance the woman's physical fitness and act as an adjunct in maintaining optimal blood glucose control. Exercise is also an excellent stress reliever. Elicit the woman's psychosocial concerns including family, job, and financial stressors and her coping mechanisms for stress.

If the woman is not familiar with techniques for self-monitoring of blood glucose, these should be taught or reviewed (see page 49). She should begin testing her blood glucose levels frequently, before meals and 1 h after meals, to assess the adequacy of her insulin regimen. Preconception goals for premeal glucose levels should be from 60 to 100 mg/dl (from 3.8 to 5.5 mmol/l), and 1-h postmeal blood glucose levels should fall to or below 120 mg/dl (≤6.7 mmol/l) (76). Based on the record of a woman's self-monitoring, the diabetes team can then prescribe adjustments in diet, insulin, or exercise that will aid her in achieving euglycemia. If the woman is adept and well motivated, she too can learn to make adjustments in her routine at home (Table 9) (73–75).

Inherent in diabetic regimens aimed at normalizing blood glucose levels is the very real risk of severe hypoglycemia (36). Before undertaking such a regimen, the woman and her partner should be warned about the risks of hypoglycemia. The educator should remind them about the signs, symptoms, and management of hypoglycemia, and the partner or a relative should be instructed in the use of glucagon. Proper education about hypoglycemia will result in fewer hospitalizations for this potentially life-threatening complication.

Serial A1C levels can be drawn monthly to confirm normalization of blood glucose levels in the preconception period. Normal or near-normal A1C levels affirm for a woman the safety of pursuing pregnancy from a metabolic standpoint (73–75). Because of interlaboratory differences in test results, the same laboratory should be used to measure A1C before and throughout pregnancy.

Finally, the woman should put into practice general principles of good health that may include cessation of smoking, alcohol intake, or unnecessary drugs.

In addition, every pregnant woman (and diabetic woman) is considered to be at higher risk for thyroid disorder and needs to have her thyroid function measured. The American Thyroid Association recommends that all women be screened for hypothyroidism during the childbearing years and that the normal range for thyroid function preconceptionally and throughout pregnancy is a free T4 of 1.0–1.6 mg/dl and a TSH in the range of 1.3–2.5 μU/l (77,78).

Although congenital anomalies and SAB are significantly increased in the offspring of a woman with preexisting diabetes, efforts to normalize blood glucose and A1C levels in the preconceptional period have resulted in a significant decrease in the incidence of congenital anomalies and SAB. Thus, any woman contemplating pregnancy will want to optimize her chances for a good outcome by enrolling in a preconception program that includes proper counseling, assessment, and management as outlined above.

PREVIOUS GDM

A woman who has had GDM in a previous pregnancy is at significant risk to develop:

- GDM in subsequent pregnancies
- Type 2 diabetes in the future

For these reasons, it is important to provide the woman with a past history of GDM with information about these associated risks. Ideally, "prepregnancy" counseling should begin in the immediate postpartum period, when a woman is still sensitive to the rigors of diabetes management.

After appropriate postpartum testing (see page 156), the woman should return for a counseling session with her physician, at which time he or she can review the results of her postpartum glucose tests with her. The physician should question her regarding her future pregnancy plans. During this visit, the physician can review the advantages and disadvantages of each method of birth control as it applies to her individual situation (see page 30).

The physician can then explain to the woman that she has an ~60–70% chance of developing GDM in future pregnancies (33). There is some suggestion that weight reduction before a future pregnancy may reduce the risk of recurrent GDM; thus, if obese, the woman should be strongly encouraged to lose weight before undertaking another pregnancy (73). During this "teachable" period, when she has just experienced the daily commitment required of a person with diabetes, she may be more motivated to follow a weight-reduction plan. If she is willing, she can then be referred for effective dietary counseling.

Finally, the woman should be encouraged to have a yearly follow-up with her physician. At this session, the physician can determine a fasting glucose level (normal value <100 mg/dl [<5.6 mmol/l]), assess success in weight reduction if appropriate, and review pregnancy plans. If there is any suspicion that diabetes has developed in the interim, the patient should be tested appropriately (see page 156). Subsequent planning for pregnancy will depend on the findings during these annual visits. Of course, if the patient has developed diabetes and desires pregnancy, she should be enrolled immediately in the prepregnancy program described above for women with preexisting diabetes (73).

REFERENCES

1. Hare JW, White P: Pregnancy in diabetes complicated by vascular disease. *Diabetes* 26:953–55, 1977

2. Jovanovic L, Druzin M, Peterson CM: Effect of euglycemia on the outcome of pregnancy in insulin dependent diabetic women as compared with normal control subjects. *Am J Med* 71:921–27, 1982

3. Coustan DR, Berkowitz RL, Hobbins JC: Tight metabolic control of overt diabetes in pregnancy. *Am J Med* 68:845–52, 1980

4. Steel JM: Prepregnancy counseling and the management of the pregnant woman with diabetes. In *Proceedings of the 39th Annual Advanced Postgraduate Course, Orlando, FL, 1992.* Alexandria, VA, American Diabetes Association, 1992, p. 97–98

5. Miodovnik M, Lavin JP, Knowles HC, Holroyde J, Stys S: Spontaneous abortion among insulin-dependent diabetic women. *Am J Obstet Gynecol* 150:372–75, 1984

6. Kitzmiller JL, Cloherty JP, Younger MD, Tabatabaii A, Rothchild S, Sosenko I, Epstein M, Sinah S, Neff R: Diabetic pregnancy and perinatal outcome. *Am J Obstet Gynecol* 131:560–80, 1978

7. Reece EA, Gabriella S, Abdalla M: The prevention of diabetes associated birth defects. *Semin Perinatol* 12:292–302, 1988

8. Reece EA, Hobbins JS: Diabetic embryopathy: pathogenesis, prenatal diagnosis and prevention. *Obstet Gynecol Surv* 41:325–35, 1986

9. Greene MF: Prevention and diagnosis of congenital anomalies in diabetic pregnancy. *Clin Perinatol* 20:533–47, 1993

10. Kalter H, Warkany J: Congenital malformations: etiologic factors and their role in prevention. *N Engl J Med* 308:424–31, 1983

11. Sadler TW, Hunter ES, Wynn RE, Phillips LH: Evidence for multifactorial origin of diabetes-induced embryopathies. *Diabetes* 38:70–74, 1989

12. Freinkel N, Lewis NJ, Akazawa S, Roth S, Forman L: The honeybee syndrome: implications of the teratogenicity of mannose in rat-embryo culture. *N Engl J Med* 310:223–30, 1984

13. Mills JL, Baker L, Goldman AS: Malformations in infants of diabetic mothers occur before the seventh gestational week: implications for treatment. *Diabetes* 28:292–93, 1979

14. Greene MF, Hare JW, Cloherty JP, Benacerraf BR, Soeldner JS: First-trimester hemoglobin A1 and risk for major malformation and spontaneous abortion in diabetic pregnancy. *Teratology* 39:225–31, 1989

15. Miller E, Hare JW, Cloherty JP, Dunn PH, Gleason RE, Soeldner JS, Kitzmiller JL: Elevated maternal hemoglobin A1c in early pregnancy and major congenital anomalies in infants of diabetic mothers. *N Engl J Med* 304:1331–34, 1981

16. Ylinen K, Aula P, Stenman U-H, Kesaniemi-Kuokkanea T, Teramo K: Risk of minor and major fetal malformations in diabetics with high haemoglobin A1c values in early pregnancy. *Br Med J* 289:345–46, 1984

17. Führmann K, Reiher H, Semmler K, Glockner E: The effect of intensified conventional insulin therapy before and during pregnancy on the malformation rate in offspring of diabetic mothers. *Exp Clin Endocrinol* 83:173–77, 1984

18. Johnstone FO, Hepburn DA, Smith AF: Can prepregnancy care of diabetic women reduce the risk of abnormal babies? *Br Med J* 301:1070–74, 1990

19. Kitzmiller JL, Gavin LA, Gin GD, Jovanovic-Peterson L, Main EK, Zigrang WD: Preconception care of diabetes: glycemic control prevents congenital anomalies. *JAMA* 265:731–36, 1991

20. Steel JM: Prepregnancy counseling and contraception in the insulin-dependent diabetic patient. *Clin Obstet Gynecol* 28:553–68, 1985

21. Elman KD, Welch RA, Frank RN, Goyert G, Sokol RJ: Diabetic retinopathy in pregnancy: a review. *Obstet Gynecol* 75:119–27, 1990

22. Loukovaara S, Immonen I, Teramo KA, Kaaja R: Progression of retinopathy during pregnancy in type 1 diabetic women treated with insulin lispro. *Diabetes Care* 26:1193–98, 2003

23. Diabetes Control and Complications Trial Research Group: Effect of pregnancy on microvascular complications in the Diabetes Control and Complications Trial. *Diabetes Care* 23:1084–91, 2000

24. Sheth BP: Does pregnancy accelerate the rate of progression of diabetic retinopathy? *Curr Diab Rep* 2:327–30, 2002

25. Henricsson M, Berntorp K, Berntorp E, Fernlund P, Sundkvist G: Progression of retinopathy after improved metabolic control in type 2 diabetic patients: relation to IGF-1 and hemostatic variables. *Diabetes Care* 22:1944–49, 1999

26. Phelps RL, Sakol P, Metzger BE, Jampol LM, Freinkel N: Changes in diabetic retinopathy during pregnancy: correlations with regulation of hyperglycemia. *Arch Ophthalmol* 104:1806–10, 1986

27. Chew EY, Mills JL, Metzger BE, Remaley NA, Jovanovic L, Knopp RH, Conley M, Rand L, Simpson JL, Holmes LB, et al.: Metabolic control and progression of retinopathy: The Diabetes in Early Pregnancy Study: National Institute of Child Health and Human Development Diabetes in Early Pregnancy Study. *Diabetes Care* 18:631–37, 1995

29. Kitzmiller JL, Main E, Ward B, Theiss T, Peterson DL: Insulin lispro and the development of proliferative diabetic retinopathy during pregnancy. *Diabetes Care* 22:874–76, 1999

30. Buchbinder A, Miodovnik M, McElvy S, Rosenn B, Kranias G, Khoury J, Siddiqi TA: Is insulin lispro associated with the development or progression of diabetic retinopathy during pregnancy? *Am J Obstet Gynecol* 183:1162–65, 2000

31. Jovanovic L: Retinopathy risk: what is responsible? Hormones, hyperglycemia, or Humalog? Response to Kitzmiller et al. *Diabetes Care* 22:846–48, 1999

32. Warram JH, Martin BC, Krowlewski AS: Risk of IDDM in children of diabetic mothers decreases with increasing maternal age at pregnancy. *Diabetes* 40:1679–84, 1991

33. American Diabetes Association: *Diabetes 1996 Vital Statistics*. Alexandria, VA, American Diabetes Association, 1996, p. 21

34. American Diabetes Association: Position statement: preconception care of women with diabetes. *Diabetes Care* 23 (Suppl. 1):S63–68, 2000

35. Chew EY, Mills JL, Metzger BE, Remaley NA, Jovanovic L, Knopp RH, Conley M, Rand L, Simpson JL, Holmes LB, Aarons JH, National Institute of Child Health and Human Development Diabetes in Early Pregnancy Study Group: Metabolic control and progression of retinopathy: The Diabetes in Early Pregnancy Study. *Diabetes Care* 18:631–37, 1995

36. Lorenz RA, Santiago JV, Siebert C, Cleary PA, Heyse S: Epidemiology of severe hypoglycemia in the Diabetes Control and Complications Trial. *Am J Med* 90:450–59, 1991

37. Philipson EH, Super DM: Gestational diabetes mellitus: does it recur in subsequent pregnancy? *Am J Obstet Gynecol* 160:1324–31, 1989

38. Hansson L, Zanchetti A, Carruthers SG, Dahlof B, Elmfeldt D, Julius S, Menard J, Rahn KH, Wedel H, Westerling S: Effects of intensive blood pressure lowering and low-dose aspirin in patients with hypertension: principal results of the Hypertension Optimal Treatment (HOT randomized trial: The HOT Study Group). *Lancet* 351:1755–62, 1998

39. UK Prospective Diabetes Study Group: Tight blood pressure control and risk of macrovascular and microvascular complications in type 2 diabetes: UKPDS 38. *BMJ* 317:703–13, 1998

40. Lazarus JM, Bourgoignie JJ, Buckalew VM, Green T, Levey AS, Milas NC, Paranandi L, Peterson JC, Porash JG, Rauch S, Soucie HM, Stollar C: Achievement and safety of a low BP goal in chronic renal disease: The Modification of Diet in Renal Disease Study Group. *Hypertension* 29:641–50, 1997

41. Arauz-Pacheco C, Parrott MA, Raskin P: The treatment of hypertension in patients with diabetes (Technical Review). *Diabetes Care* 25:134–47, 2002

42. American Diabetes Association: Hypertension management in adults with diabetes. *Diabetes Care* 27:S65–67, 2005

43. Bakris GL, Williams M, Dworkin L, Elliott, WJ, Epstein M, Toto R, Tuttle K, Douglas J, Hsueh W, Sowers J, for the National Kidney Foundation Hypertension and Diabetes Executive Committees Working Group: Preserving renal function in adults with hypertension and diabetes: a consensus approach. *Am J Kidney Dis* 36:646–61, 2000

44. World Health Organization: *The Hypertensive Disorders of Pregnancy.* Geneva, World Health Organization, Tech. Rep. Ser., no. 758, 1987, p. 8–15

45. Von Dadelszen P, Ornstein MP, Bull SB, Logan AG, Koren G, Magee LA: Fall in mean arterial pressure and fetal growth restriction in pregnancy hypertension: a meta-analysis. *Lancet* 355:87–92, 2000

46. Ochsenbein-Kolble N, Roos M, Gasser T, Huch R, Zimmermann R: Cross sectional study of automated blood pressure measurements throughout pregnancy. *Br J Obstet Gynaecol* 111:319–25, 2004

47. Peterson CM, Jovanovic-Peterson L, Mills JL, Conley MR, Knopp RH, Reed GF, Aarons JH, Holmes LB, Brown Z, Van Allen M, Schmeltz R, Metzger BE, the National Institute of Child Health and Human Development–The

Diabetes in Early Pregnancy Study: Changes in cholesterol, triglycerides, body weight, and blood pressure. *Am J Obstet Gynecol* 166:513–18, 1992

48. Biesenbach G, Grafinger P, Stoger H, Zarzgornik J 2nd: How pregnancy influences renal function in nephropathic type 1 diabetic women depends on their pre-conceptional creatinine clearance. *J Nephrol* 12:41–46, 1999

49. Briggs GG, Freeman RK, Yaffe SJ, Eds. *Drugs in Pregnancy and Lactation.* 6th ed. Philadelphia, Lippincott Williams & Wilkins, 2002

50. Saji H, Yamanaka M, Hagiwara A, Ijiri F: Losartan and fetal toxic effects. *Lancet* 357:363, 2001

51. Lepore M, Pampanelli S, Fanelli C, Porcellati F, Bartocci L, Di Vincenzo A, Cordoni C, Costa E, Brunetti P, Bolli GM: Pharmacokinetics and pharmaco-dynamics of subcutaneous injection of long-acting human insulin analog glargine, NPH insulin and ultralente human insulin and continuous subcuta-neous infusion of insulin lispro. *Diabetes* 49:2142–48, 2000

52. Bolli GB, Perriello G, Fanelli C, De Feo P: Nocturnal blood glucose control in type 1 diabetes mellitus. *Diabetes Care* 16 (Suppl. 3):71–89, 1993

53. Lindstrom T, Olsson PO, Arnqvist HJ: The use of human ultralente is limited by great intraindividual variability in overnight plasma insulin profiles. *Scand J Clin Lab Invest* 60:341–47, 2000

54. Kimmerle R, Heinemann L, Delecki A, Berger M: Severe hypoglycemia: incidence and predisposing factors in 85 pregnancies of type 1 diabetic women. *Diabetes Care* 15:1034–37, 1992

55. Evers IM, deValk HW, Visser GHA: Risk of complications of pregnancy in women with type 1 diabetes: nationwide prospective study in the Nether-lands. *BMJ* 328:915, 2004

56. Anderson JH Jr, Brunelle RL, Koivisto VA, Pfützner A, Trautmann ME, Vig-nati L, DiMarchi R: Reduction of postprandial hyperglycemia and frequency of hypoglycemia in IDDM patients on insulin-analog treatment: Multicenter Insulin Lispro Study Group. *Diabetes* 46:265–70, 1997

57. Del Sindaco P, Ciofetta M, Lalli C, Perriello G, Pampanelli S, Torlone E, Brunetti P, Bolli GB: Use of the short-acting insulin analogue lispro in inten-sive treatment of type 1 diabetes mellitus: importance of appropriate replace-ment of basal insulin and time-interval injection-meal. *Diabet Med* 15:592–600, 1998

58. Ebeling P, Jansson PA, Smith U, Lalli C, Bolli GB, Koivisto VA: Strategies toward improved control during insulin lispro therapy in IDDM: importance of basal insulin. *Diabetes Care* 20:1287–89, 1997

59. Brunelle BL, Llewelyn J, Anderson JH Jr, Gale EA, Koivisto VA: Meta-analy-sis of the effect of insulin lispro on severe hypoglycemia in patients with type 1 diabetes. *Diabetes Care* 21:1726–31, 1998

60. Colombel A, Murat A, Krempf M, Kuchly-Anton B, Charbonnel B: Improve-ment of blood glucose control in type 1 diabetic patients treated with lispro and multiple NPH injections. *Diabet Med* 16:319–24, 1999

61. Wyatt JW, Frias JL, Hoyme HE, Jovanovic L, Kaaja R, Brown F, Garg S, Lee-Parritz A, Seely EW, Kerr L, Mattoo V, Tan M, IONS study group: Congenital anomaly rate in offspring of mothers with type 1 diabetes treated with insulin lispro during pregnancy. *Diabet Med* 21:2001–07, 2004

62. Garg SK, Frias JP, Anil S, Gottlieb PA, Mackenzie T, Jackson WE: Insulin lispro therapy in pregnancies complicated by diabetes type 1: glycemic control and maternal and fetal outcomes. *Endocr Pract* 9:187–93, 2003

63. Masson EA, Patmore JE, Brash PD, Baxter M, Caldwell G, Gallen AW, Price PA, Vice PA, Walker JD, Lindow SW: Pregnancy outcome in type 1 diabetes mellitus treated with insulin lispro (Humalog). *Diabet Med* 20:46–50, 2003

64. Bhattacharyya A, Brown S, Hughes S, Vice PA: Insulin lispro and regular insulin in pregnancy. *QJM* 94:255–60, 2001

65. Idama TO, Lindow SW, French M, Masson EA: Preliminary experience with the use of insulin lispro in pregnant diabetic women. *J Obstet Gynecol* 21:350–51, 2001

66. Persson B, Swahn M, Hjertberg R, Hanson U, Nord E, Nordlander E, Hansson LO: Insulin lispro therapy in pregnancies complicated by type 1 diabetes mellitus. *Diabetes Res Clin Pract* 58:115–21, 2002

67. Loukovaara S, Immonen I, Teramo KA, Kaaja R: Progression of retinopathy during pregnancy in type 1 diabetic women treated with insulin lispro. *Diabetes Care* 26:1193–98, 2003

68. Jovanovic L, Ilic S, Pettitt DJ, Hugo K, Gutierrez M, Bowsher RR, Bastyr EJ 3rd: Metabolic and immunologic effects of insulin lispro in gestational diabetes. *Diabetes Care* 22:1422–27, 1999

69. Pettitt DJ, Ospina P, Kolaczynski JW, Jovanovic L: Comparison of an insulin analog, insulin aspart, and regular human insulin with no insulin in gestational diabetes mellitus. *Diabetes Care* 26:183–86, 2003

70. Mecacci F, Carignani L, Cioni R, Bartoli E, Parretti E, La Torre P, Scarselli G, Mello G: Maternal metabolic control and perinatal outcome in women with gestational diabetes treated with regular or lispro insulin: comparison with non-diabetic pregnant women. *Eur J Obste Bynecol Reprod Biol* 111:19–24, 2003

71. Kurtzhals P, Schaffer L, Sorensen A, Kristensen C, Jonassen I, Schmid C, Trüb T: Correlations of receptor binding and metabolic and mitogenic potencies of insulin analogs designed for clinical use. *Diabetes* 49:999–1005, 2000

72. Ciaraldi TP, Carter L, Seipke G, Mudaliar S, Henry RR: Effects of the long-acting insulin glargine on cultured human skeletal muscle cells: comparisons to insulin and IGF-1. *J Clin Endocrinol Metab* 86:5838, 2001

73. American Diabetes Association: Nutrition recommendations and principles for people with diabetes mellitus (Position Statement). *Diabetes Care* 23 (Suppl. 1):S43–46, 2000

74. Jovanovic L, Peterson CM, Saxena BB, Dawood MY, Saudek CD: Feasibility of maintaining euglycemia in insulin-dependent diabetic women. *Am J Med* 68:105–12, 1980

75. Jovanovic L, Druzin M, Peterson CM: The effect of euglycemia on the outcome of pregnancy in insulin-dependent diabetics as compared to normal controls. *Am J Med* 71:921–27, 1981

76. Jovanovic L, Peterson CM, Reed GF, Metzger BE, Mills JL, Knopp RH, Aarons JH: Maternal postprandial glucose levels and infant birth weight: the Diabetes in Early Pregnancy Study: The National Institute of Child Health and Human Development–Diabetes in Early Pregnancy Study. *Am J Obstet Gynecol* 164:103–11, 1991

77. American Thyroid Association: Consensus Statement #2: American Thyroid Association statement on early maternal thyroidal insufficiency: recognition, clinical management and research directions. *Thyroid* 15:77–79, 2005

78. Jovanovic L, Peterson CM: De novo hypothyroidism in pregnancies complicated by type I diabetes and proteinuria: a new syndrome. *Am J Obstet Gynecol* 159:441–46, 1988

Contraction

Highlights
Contraception

■ Contraceptive counseling is an effective method for avoiding the undesirable consequences of an unplanned diabetic pregnancy. No one contraceptive method is appropriate for all women with diabetes, and counseling must be individualized.

■ If an oral contraceptive is the best choice, a combined or sequential pill with ≤35 μg estrogen and a low progestin dose may be best, but the risk of cardiovascular effects must be considered. Progestin-only pills offer an alternative, but there is the possibility of elevated blood lipid levels and other effects.

■ Use of the long-acting injectable progestin is no longer recommended for diabetic patients.

■ Copper-containing intrauterine devices appear to expose diabetic women to no greater risk of infection than they do to nondiabetic women.

■ Once childbearing is completed, permanent sterilization of the diabetic woman or her mate may offer an acceptable means to prevent unplanned pregnancy compared with other contraceptive methods.

Contraception

Hen a prescription for contraception is given to the patient with diabetes, the health care provider must consider not only the general risks and benefits of a particular mode of contraception but also the potential risks that are specific to diabetes. However, it is equally important to consider the consequences, both medical and social, of an unplanned pregnancy. Should pregnancy occur in the presence of poor metabolic control, the likelihood of major congenital anomalies in the offspring is increased markedly. The successful completion of a "high-risk" pregnancy is expensive and labor intensive; part of prepregnancy planning should involve an assessment of health insurance coverage, as well as consideration of the social support system that will be necessary for the patient to adhere to an appointment and testing schedule and to have help readily available should unanticipated problems, such as hypoglycemic reactions or hospitalization, occur. If the patient already has one or more children, it is important to plan for help with child care during the pregnancy. For these reasons, contraception is an important topic to be discussed with any woman who has diabetes.

Women with the previous diagnosis of gestational diabetes mellitus (GDM) but who currently have documented normal glucose metabolism theoretically do not have the same increased risk of vascular disease as do women with type 1 or type 2 diabetes. Nevertheless, close to 40–60% of women with previous GDM will develop diabetes within 20 yr of their index pregnancy, so that the same general considerations should be taken into account as for women with preexisting diabetes.

There is no single contraceptive method appropriate for all women with diabetes. Each has advantages and drawbacks (Table 10). Therefore, the most commonly available methods are discussed individually. Contraceptive efficacy should always be assessed in relation to the pregnancy rate for sexual activity with no protection, which is ~85% in a year's exposure.

ORAL CONTRACEPTIVES

Oral contraceptives are available as combined (estrogen plus progestin), progestin-only, or sequential (often called triphasic) formulations. Although the first combined preparations available, containing rather high doses of steroid compounds, were associated with increasing insulin resistance, commonly available low-dose preparations have not been associated with significant deterioration of glucose metabolism and are probably safe for individuals with diabetes from the

Table 10   Contraceptive Methods for Diabetic Women

Type	Effectiveness (%)	Disadvantages
Oral contraceptives		
Low-dose combined (estrogen + progestin) or sequential ethinyl estradiol + new progestin (levonorgestrel, desogestrel, gestodene, or norgestimate)	98	Oral agent of choice if ethinyl estradiol is <35 µg in combination with new progestin
Progestin only	94	May increase serum lipids and glucose levels
Barrier methods		
Diaphragm + spermicide	82	High failure rate
Condom + foam	88	High failure rate; prevents some sexually transmitted diseases
Rhythm	80	Diabetic women may not have regular menstrual cycles,thus increasing failure rate
Sterilization	99+	Essentially irreversible

standpoint of glycemic control.

However, the estrogen compounds in combined oral contraceptives, and presumably in sequentials, have been statistically associated with increases in the risk of thromboembolism, stroke, and myocardial infarction, particularly in older women and those who smoke cigarettes. Combined oral contraceptives are best avoided by women who smoke and/or are ≥35 yr of age. Because diabetes carries a risk of vascular disease, some clinicians prefer not to prescribe combined oral contraceptives for diabetic women. Hypertension, another risk associated with diabetes, is also considered a contraindication. To minimize these risks, formulations that contain ≤35 µg estradiol and a low progestin dosage are recommended. Because estrogen raises and progesterone depresses high-density lipoprotein levels, the formulation should have estrogen predominance.

Currently used oral contraceptives containing the new progestin (levonorgestrel, desogestrel, gestodene, or norgestimate) are all classified as low dose because they all contain <35 µg ethinyl estradiol. Despite their low steroid content, they are all proven to be highly effective. The new progestins have minimal or no impact on glucose control and are not associated with an increased risk of impaired glucose tolerance. Thus, these oral contraceptives emerge as the steroid contraceptives of choice (1–3).

Progestin-only pills do not carry so great a risk of thromboembolic and vascular disease. However, these formulations are believed to be somewhat less effective than combined pills and may be associated with elevated lipid levels, glucose elevation, and irregular uterine bleeding. Progestin-only pills are therefore a problem for women who previously had GDM. In addition, the use of the long-acting injectable progestin depomedroxyprogesterone acetate (DMPA) has been reported to increase the risk of type 2 diabetes in women with previous GDM. An observational cohort study of 526 Hispanic women with prior GDM who were not diabetic in their first postpartum visit were followed up to 9.2 years, and the rate of annual diabetes incidence rates was 19% as opposed to 12% in a similar cohort of women who were taking oral contraceptives. DMPA use was associated with a significant increase in weight and elevated triglyceride levels. Thus, DMPA should be avoided when possible in women at risk for diabetes or who have diabetes (4).

BARRIER METHODS

The diaphragm has the tremendous advantage that it carries no medical risks. If a couple is highly motivated and uses a diaphragm and spermicidal jelly regularly, the method has a theoretical effectiveness as high as 98%, but "user failures" lower this effectiveness to ~85%.

Unfortunately, the diaphragm and spermicide are viewed by some couples as an intrusion into their lovemaking, and the necessity for advance planning is sometimes considered to interfere with spontaneity. Patients should be reminded that the diaphragm can be inserted 1 h before it will be needed, so that foreplay need not be interrupted. The diaphragm should be left in place for 8 h after coitus.

Diaphragm and spermicide are often chosen by women with diabetes who want to delay childbearing or space out their family and are not ready for permanent methods of sterilization. It is of the utmost importance that diaphragms be fitted by an experienced health care professional and that the patient be carefully instructed in its use.

Condom and spermicidal foam constitute another barrier method of contraception. Effectiveness is comparable with that of the diaphragm, and this method also appears to offer protection against a number of sexually transmitted diseases.

RHYTHM

Also known as physiological fertility control, the rhythm method utilizes knowledge of cyclic changes in physiology to identify the time of ovulation, so that coitus can be avoided. This approach assumes that ovulation occurs ~14 days before the onset of the next menstrual period, and that sperm survive for 48–72 h after ejaculation. It also assumes that the patient's past menstrual history can be used to calculate a "window" when ovulation is most likely to occur. Many couples also plot basal body temperatures daily to assess (retrospectively) the time of ovulation. Changes in the character of cervical mucus can also be helpful. Effectiveness is usually reported as ~75%, making this method highly unreliable and useful only to those strongly committed to the avoidance of other artificial means of contraception. It is not recommended for women with type 1 diabetes, because pregnancy should be planned in these individuals to coincide with optimal metabolic control. The high failure rate makes such planning problematic.

PERMANENT STERILIZATION

For the individual with diabetes who has completed childbearing, permanent surgical sterilization of either the woman or her mate offers a reasonable contraceptive option. It is of course necessary for the couple to be counseled as to the relative irreversibility of the procedure. Clearly, there are risks associated with any surgery, and sterilization is no exception. However, many couples find that this one-time risk is more acceptable than the daily risk of pregnancy with other methods. The pregnancy rate after surgical sterilization of the woman (or man) is <0.5%. However, those pregnancies that do occur in sterilized women are more likely to be ectopically implanted.

REFERENCES

1. Nessa A, Latif SA, Siddiqui NI: Risk of cardiovascular diseases with oral contraceptives. *Mymensingh Med J* 15:220–24, 2006

2. ACOG Committee on Practice Bulletin No. 73: Use of hormonal contraception in women with coexisting medical conditions. *Obstet Gynecol* 107:1453–72, 2006

3. Schwarz EB, Maselli J, Gonzales R: Contraceptive counseling of diabetic women of reproductive age. *Obstet Gynecol* 107:1070–74, 2006

4. Xiang AH, Lawakubo, Kjos SL, Buchanan TA: Long-acting injectable progestin contraception and risk of type 2 diabetes in Latino women with prior gestational diabetes. *Diabetes Care* 29:613–17, 2006

Psychological Impact of Diabetes and Pregnancy

Highlights
Psychological Impact of
Diabetes and Pregnancy

■ All women go through adjustment stages during their pregnancy, but these are magnified by the diabetes response to the pregnant state.

■ The emotional impact of being pregnant and managing diabetes increases stress levels.

■ Open communication between patient and clinician requires mutual respect, honesty, and cooperation. Open-ended questions provide more information. Condemning noncompliance will not lead to discovering reasons for it.

■ The patient is the final decision-maker in handling her day-to-day management. Get her involved to the best of her ability in problem solving and decision making.

■ A psychosocial assessment can provide valuable information about the patient's lifestyle, family, job, and economic situation. This can assist in providing advice that will be followed.

■ Emotional support is essential for the patient's well-being, whatever the source—spouse, other family members, health care professionals, peers, or support groups.

■ Patients with type 1 diabetes have an increased awareness of complications. Patients with type 2 diabetes focus concern on whether they will have to continue on insulin after delivery.

■ Concern about having a normal, healthy child and/or neonatal morbidity is magnified for the pregnant diabetic woman.

■ High anxiety and fear affect adherence to the pregnancy regimen for tight blood glucose control and dietary compliance. Discussion is essential to assist the patient.

■ Fear tactics do not always improve patient compliance as much as increase denial and communications breakdown. The intensity of following a strict protocol emotionally lengthens the pregnancy time span for even the most cooperative patient.

■ Prepregnancy counseling is vital for any diabetic woman of childbearing age, beginning with adolescence.

Psychological Impact of Diabetes and Pregnancy

Pregnancy is a time of physical and emotional fluctuation for any woman. However, what is true for any woman becomes intensified for a diabetic woman, who is faced with increasing demands and scrutiny regarding fetal development, managing her diabetes as it responds to the pregnancy, and increased medical management. Experienced clinicians are aware of how the emotional impact of being pregnant coupled with managing diabetes can increase stress levels for the patient.

Each woman reacts to the diagnosis of diabetes based on her established habits and family/cultural patterns of managing health, which are determined in part by her personality and learned coping methods. Most women have conflicting emotions regarding their diabetes, and even with a wanted pregnancy, they may feel ambivalent.

A myth has developed in our society that everyone should be delighted by the anticipation of having a child. Unfortunately, this illusion sometimes obscures reality. Pregnancy has several major implications for a woman: her role must expand from being responsible for just herself and relationship with her mate to including a totally dependent infant; changing body image, involving discomfort at times; a surrender of some amount of her personal freedom for an unspecified period of time; and a commitment of 18–20 yr to raising and providing for a child.

When this myth about pregnancy meets reality, a woman's thinking can change as she begins to confront the commitment she is expected to make. Some women feel guilty for having negative feelings they believe are inappropriate. Assurance from her health care professionals that such feelings are not unusual can be comforting to a woman. Her physician needs to judge whether poor blood glucose control and nonadherence are signals of ambivalence about the pregnancy or a desire to abort or miscarry. It is important not to lose sight of the fact that the only thing all people with diabetes have in common is an elevated blood glucose level.

RESPONSE TO PREGNANCY IN WOMEN WITH PREEXISTING DIABETES

Most people with diabetes live with some degree of anxiety about their disease, which they deal with in various ways: denial, rationalization, intellectualization, compulsive control, depression, and existential or fatalistic attitude. For a diabetic woman who becomes pregnant, the natural anxieties related to having diabetes can intensify depending on how well educated she is about her diabetes and what she has been told about bearing and raising children.

She may see her role of child-bearer as a way to prove her self-worth and femininity and her ability to produce a healthy, normal child. These attitudes may increase in importance if she feels some degree of depression related to having diabetes or if she has experienced a previous miscarriage or fetal demise. If the pregnancy is unwanted, negative feelings become intensified, and the potential for residual guilt along with relief increases if the pregnancy is lost, particularly when medical advice has not been followed. In addition, if the advice is that a miscarriage may occur if intensified self-care is not undertaken, then a woman who does not want the pregnancy may use this advice to fulfill a wish to have an abortion.

It is not unusual for a woman with diabetes to have been told never to bear a child. This misinformation is usually given by a health care professional who is not aware of the advances in the management of diabetic pregnancy. A woman who has been so misinformed will have increased concern about her risk of developing complications and fears that she may not live long enough to raise her child. In a survey of preconception counseling of 69 diabetic women, 18 were multiparous, and a large proportion of the diabetic women (85%) reported that they knew that their diabetes could affect the health of the baby and good diabetic control was important at the time of conception. The diabetic clinic staff provided ~60% of the advice on preconception glucose control, whereas the other advice came from leaflets or pamphlets. Only 4.5% reported that they heard the advice from "diabetes associations" (1). In another study (2), knowledge about preconception care in French women with type 1 diabetes was assessed. Data for all type 1 diabetic women in 11 diabetes centers were included. An anonymous dual questionnaire was administered. A total of 138 women were included. The main source of advice about preconception care was noted to be from the physician, and 42% responded that they obtained the advice from a pamphlet. However, 48% claimed that they were unaware of the risk of congenital anomalies related to their blood glucose control, and 41% feared that their baby would be born with diabetes manifesting in the neonatal period. Thus, despite admitting that advice was given about preconception glucose control, the majority of type 1 diabetic women have a major knowledge deficit concerning the risks associated with pregnancy. The observation that we have not been successful in preconception education is at least a first step to solving the problem (2).

Because maintaining normal blood glucose levels before becoming pregnant seems to lower the risk of birth anomalies, make this reassuring information available to patients of childbearing age. Pregnant patients should also understand that blood glucose levels can fluctuate regardless of complete adherence to the protocol. In addition, the myth that increased insulin dosages equal worsening diabetes needs to be dismissed: increased insulin dosage is expected as the placenta grows. Type 2 diabetic patients whose prepregnancy diabetes is controlled without insulin but who require insulin injections for normal blood glucose control during pregnancy may be concerned about whether they will remain on insulin after delivery (1–3).

RESPONSE TO THE DIAGNOSIS OF GESTATIONAL DIABETES

Nutritional counseling is a priority for the gestational diabetic woman. Her education should include information about what gestational diabetes is and why it can occur in pregnancy, the reason for frequent blood and urine testing, and the possibility that insulin may be required later in the pregnancy.

Women with gestational diabetes are not only coping emotionally with the pregnancy but are also confronted with a potentially life-threatening health problem that will become intensified if they are placed on an insulin regimen. The natural anxieties of pregnancy and the fear that they will have to remain on insulin after delivery increase. These fears can affect the ability of the woman with gestational diabetes to learn the necessary daily fundamentals of diabetes management. Personal and cultural health beliefs about diabetes, taking insulin, and why this disease occurred can also affect her ability to learn. In a study of women referred to the California Diabetes and Pregnancy Sweet Success Program between June 2001 and 2003, analysis was undertaken to estimate the risk of macrosomia. Compared with college-educated women, women without a college education were 35% more likely to deliver a macrosomic infant. Thus, gestational diabetes in a woman with a lower level of education appears to have an increased risk of macrosomia (4). Reinforcement and repetition of information are important. However, the need for repetition is not necessarily a sign of an inherent problem in learning self-care. It is not unusual for an anxious patient to retain only one-third of what is originally taught about diabetes care due to blocking. Some women with gestational diabetes also feel increased ambivalence toward the developing baby. If the diabetes continues after delivery, hostility toward the child, who might be seen as the cause of the diabetes, may be provoked.

LONG-TERM ADAPTATION

It is generally difficult to convince anyone that current behavioral changes are important for their continued long-term well-being. Human nature tends to resist change, and when it is required, people look for short-term success. However, permanent behavioral change is not possible unless the individual experiences an attitudinal shift within herself to make the commitment to change her behavior. Even then, permanent behavioral change can take from 6 mo to 2 yr.

Adapting to the demands of diabetes means changes in lifestyle and daily choices. Diabetes affects spontaneity and relationships with significant others in regard to eating habits, exercise, and self-care. Proper diabetes care takes extra time, thought, preplanning, and other things not usually considered by the non-diabetic person. How well a woman adjusts is affected by prior life experiences and present occurrences in her life as well as her personality, family support (or lack of it), and ways of coping with stress and crisis.

Diabetes education walks a fine line between hope and reality. It is important to support a positive perspective by trying to encourage patients to "slot" the diabetes as just one facet of their life, not the be-all and the end-all. Making a priority list can help point out that life is more than diabetes and that "healthy denial" is valuable because it enables a person with diabetes to cope in a realistic way rather than be burdened with anxiety and depression.

Marked fluctuations in blood glucose levels affect mental and emotional states. It is not much of a quantum jump for some people to fear that diabetes is driving them crazy, particularly if they do not suspect the interrelationship between physiological and psychological body chemistry that research is revealing. Although some degree of mild depression and anxiety is not unusual in diabetes due to its chronicity and potential long-term complications, it need not be uppermost in a person's mind.

An important motivating factor for a pregnant diabetic woman is remaining healthy to raise her child. The health care professional's approach is a vital guide in structuring a patient's emotional perspective about herself and her diabetes. The diabetes lifestyle is healthy for everyone. If she can make the commitment to live as balanced a life as possible within the requirements the diabetes establishes, her reward will be feeling healthy and well balanced rather than plagued by illness, fatigue, anxiety, and depression.

PERSONALITY TYPES AND INDIVIDUALIZING TREATMENT

Numerous studies have revealed that no typical diabetic personality exists (5). Individuals with various personality types make up the diabetic population, each with different maturity and intelligence levels and established patterns of coping with the complexities of diabetes and, in this instance, pregnancy.

It is essential to individualize treatment as much as possible to enable the patient to maximize adaptation to a diabetic pregnancy. Taking a psychosocial history is a good first step. Patients are human beings first; having diabetes does not create perfection, although some health care professionals expect it.

Yet another diabetes myth fostered by clinicians is that, if the patient follows her diabetes treatment plan, her body will respond appropriately. Realistically, diabetes does not always respond to current treatment methodologies. Not only are there many causes for fluctuating blood glucose levels, but patients differ in the level of interest in their condition and treatment as well as capacity for understanding diabetes and accepting and applying information. By becoming sensitive to the variations in patients' needs at different stages in their pregnancy, the clinician becomes more effective in enhancing patient adaptation to the diabetes regimen (6).

The following personality definitions describe the possible psychological profiles a clinician may find in the practice setting, with recommendations for management.

COMPULSIVE PERSON

Attitude: This patient is orderly, controlled with management, and knowledgeable about diabetes and its effects on the body and appears self-disciplined; her driving motivation is related to underlying anxiety of having diabetes.

Response to management: This patient is cooperative when treated as an equal; her anxiety level increases when the diabetes does not respond to "perfect" care, with anger toward clinicians if their management is not as rigid as hers. Hospitalization may be difficult because of her having to surrender her independence.

Management approach: Make her an active team member with care, decision making, and options; support active participation in self-care; keep her well informed, with discussion and clear communication; give her reassurances that diabetes in pregnancy functions differently than in a nonpregnant state.

IMMATURE PERSON

Attitude: This patient's attitude is inconsistent with management. She exhibits strong denial (disavowing the diabetes), rebellion, anger, resentment, regressive behavior to a younger age level, and childishness.

Response to management: This patient has difficulty adhering to the regimen and regularity; dietary indiscretion is common, as is failure to keep appointments and records, refusal to alter lifestyle to any significant degree, hostility toward health care providers, and potential for a reactive depression if denial is dismantled.

Management approach: Use a firm, supportive, nonpunitive manner; use patience; help her recognize that the ability to have control to make decisions is beneficial to herself and her baby. Notice and encourage any positive effort, no matter how small, to follow the regimen; avoid overcriticism. Comment on dissatisfaction with her behavior and not with her as a person.

HYSTERICAL PERSON

Attitude: This patient is dramatic, emotional, overanxious, and fearful and exhibits strong feelings of being defective secondary to having diabetes.

Response to management: This patient watches for the clinician's level of involvement with her case, fears rejection, and worries about regimen and procedures.

Management approach: Be consistent and firm, and give continuing reassurance about interest in her case. Focus on her capacity to help herself and what she can do (to help relieve some anxiety and fear).

DEMANDING DEPENDENT PERSON

Attitude: This patient has difficulty with self-management when not pregnant, expects others to care for her diabetes, is petulant and helpless, demands attention, and has deep-seated dependency needs that are not being met.

Response to management: This patient wants to be taken care of and have others make all decisions, resists taking responsibility, and seeks extra attention.

Management approach: Set reasonable limits within the support offered, communicate and demonstrate interest in her well-being with attention to detail, make telephone contact and extra appointments available if deemed necessary, and praise her for any responsible effort. Cooperation may improve if care is shared by her mate or other family member.

MASOCHISTIC PERSON

Attitude: This patient has a low self-image and diminished self-esteem; she feels she deserves bad luck and may have chronic depression.

Response to management: This patient expects misfortune and things to go wrong and may have difficulty following through with the regimen on her own behalf. Depression may limit her ability to learn and apply what is taught; she may chronically complain despite adequate treatment.

Management approach: Give consistent support, suggest she follow the regimen for her baby or others if she is unable to do it for herself, show continued interest, and give reassurance and encouragement.

PASSIVE DEPENDENT PERSON

Attitude: This patient wants others to make decisions for her, lacks self-worth, has difficulty making decisions, yields to others' choices, and is submissive.

Response to management: She resists taking responsibility or decision making so she cannot be blamed if things do not work, relies on others for support, and may have difficulty acting on recommendations.

Management approach: Provide continued support and telephone contact when appointments are not kept and ongoing encouragement and recognition for any efforts with her regimen; enlist help from any support source—mate, family, friends, or agency.

In a study of 100 patients, psychiatric risk factors in diabetic pregnancy were revealed as follows: adolescent pregnancy; previous psychiatric treatment; marital problems; single parenthood; concurrent medical illness (other than diabetes); a history of two or more spontaneous abortions or stillbirths; age >35 yr; obesity; and low socioeconomic status (7). All these factors were overrepresented in women with psychological disturbance.

DEALING WITH CRISES

HOSPITALIZATION

Being admitted to the hospital can increase the stress levels for the pregnant diabetic woman unless she can view it as an acceptable escape from a difficult situation. Some clinicians realize that hospitalization for blood glucose control is not always realistic, because the patient is no longer functioning in a normal environment, and the separation from her family may create an additional strain.

With the availability of blood glucose self-monitoring and a team approach providing support and encouragement, many patients develop an enhanced sense of self-control when managing the situation in their own environment. The informed, motivated patient may demonstrate ambivalence during a prolonged hospital stay if she is feeling well and becoming restless and bored by the limited activity. She may also resent others making decisions about her health management, particularly if she is excluded from discussions, removed from self-responsibility, and not allowed to share her opinion when she has been able to manage her regimen well at home.

Appropriate dayroom or patio privileges, exercise, and involving the patient in treatment discussions should be allowed to help maintain a balance in her life. The more dependent, less mature patient may enjoy the additional attention she receives during a hospitalization and be quite willing for the staff to take over her diabetes care. She needs limits and encouragement to participate in her management when it is feasible.

FETAL DEMISE

Most women at some point in their pregnancy have some awareness of the possibility of a miscarriage. This anxiety is particularly intensified in the diabetic patient. For the woman who very much wants a child, such awareness can increase her anxiety and fear of something happening to her baby. Ordinarily, such anxiety in nondiabetic women is suppressed and superseded by the anticipation of a healthy child.

A woman's response to a fetal loss is determined by several factors: her socio-cultural-religious beliefs, the strength of her commitment to have a child, her personality, and her coping capacities in handling loss. There is a psychological as well as physical sense of loss because the experience reinforces her feelings of a lack of normalcy, further damaging her self-image and feminine self-esteem. The anxiety and fear level, already present to some degree, now becomes grounded in reality because her primary feminine function, to produce a healthy child, has been undermined, and she perceives herself as having failed in that role. She is not only threatened by this complication but also fearful of her capacity to reproduce. Expressions of guilt from not having done certain things related to the regimen dictated by the diabetes are not unusual. If she has followed the regimen to the best of her ability, she can be bitter and angry because she feels the effort she made and the limitations she endured did not matter.

Grieving is a natural and necessary reaction to all types of loss. It enables a person to recognize the finality of the loss and to integrate feelings and thoughts in a healthy way. Increased anxiety is generated by a loss of control over one's life functioning. A fear of potential rejection and abandonment by her partner may exist. Some women become depressed because of anger turned inward and generated by self-blame, rejection of the imperfect self, and loss of the illusion of invulnerability and omnipotence. This depression is not an unnatural response; the woman has been frustrated and deprived of her goal to have a healthy child. Her depression is a reflection of a realistically unpleasant event that led to an understandable sadness. The symptoms of her sadness may not be consistent and may demonstrate a wavelike quality that increases or recedes at different times.

At such a time, the support of health care professionals as empathetic listeners should not be underestimated. This healing dimension provides a supportive baseline to the patient with her own healing by providing a sense of participation in living and managing the grieving process. Facilitating the grieving process represents a vital part of caring. It encompasses one's simple presence and availability as a nonjudgmental, receptive listener who accepts and legitimizes the woman's right to her emotions while providing an avenue for their expression when she is ready to do so. Effective management encourages the woman to face her fears and anxiety about a future pregnancy. The expression of such feelings not only assists with her grieving and diminishes denial but can also help her learn to handle any sense of helplessness and/or hopelessness. The relationship should be maintained at a level that enables her to talk freely and express any feelings.

It is of value to discern the emotional health of the patient and how it relates to her needs. This assessment can be determined not only from the patient but also from her family, other staff members, and her history. It is also beneficial to be cognizant of her religious beliefs regarding treatment, family situation, and support system or lack of it. This awareness can enable the clinician to initiate interventions to assist the patient and her family in meeting their needs. Another consideration may be to share information regarding the prospect of a future pregnancy or possible adoption.

CONGENITAL ANOMALIES

The woman who delivers an infant with a congenital anomaly may have feelings similar to the patient experiencing a fetal loss or stillbirth. The distinct difference is being confronted with having a child with medical problems, which creates a sense of shock and disbelief. Although the risk of delivering a child with medical problems is known, most people tend to believe that such things happen only to others. The feelings involved with delivering such a baby may last from a few days to years. On a deeper level, there are feelings of hurt pride, wrongdoing, defectiveness, and diminished self-esteem and self-worth.

These emotions need to be handled in a supportive and noncritical manner to enhance healthy self-esteem and encourage a positive attitude for handling the child's condition in a realistic way. It is important to observe and encourage bonding between the mother and her infant. For the most effective bonding to occur, she should be allowed to touch and be with her baby even if the infant is critically ill. Studies have shown that mothers of critically ill or stillborn infants resolve their grieving more rapidly when given the opportunity to be with and hold their baby (8). She will eventually require referral to community agencies that can assist and provide services for her and her child.

THE IMPORTANCE OF A TEAM APPROACH

With rapidly expanding medical technology and knowledge, health care specialization is increasing, often at the cost of diminished human interaction between health care professionals and their patients. Because of the complexity of diabetes, a patient can be involved with numerous clinicians. Effective interdisciplinary communication enhances the collaborative effort on the patient's behalf for a successful pregnancy outcome (9).

It is important to realize that the patient is the final decision-maker in following the advice given and needs to be included whenever feasible in planning her diabetes and pregnancy care. If a problem exists for her in doing so, workable solutions should be implemented after exploring her particular needs. Any discussion with the pregnant patient should encompass the unique role and responsibilities she will have in the management of her pregnancy that differ from the traditional model of the physician having the full responsibility (10). Such an approach can help a woman feel more in control of her daily life, which decreases the potential for hospitalization.

Group discussions and one-on-one counseling with a clinical social worker or psychologist and other patients can provide emotional support and psychosocial problem interventions. It also affords the patient an opportunity for attitudinal change and maturational growth regarding her beliefs about health care, her own maternal/feminine roles, coping options, and herself.

Pregnancy can provide an ideal opportunity for teaching aimed at motivating the patient in improved long-term diabetes management. Educational information can be provided verbally, and printed materials and audiovisual formats are available on diabetes and pregnancy, exercise, breastfeeding, childbirth, sterilization, birth control, postpartum care, and parenting.

Many patients find that, if they are given the responsibility as an equal participant in their care, it is a new health care management approach for them. It is not unusual for them to be somewhat doubtful initially that they can take this responsibility in the light of prior experiences until they actually see the clinician using such a concept. Even with difficult-to-manage patients, there can be a positive attitudinal effect if they are made to feel in control. Treated as a responsible adult and as the unique individual she is, a patient can respond and adapt to the demanding regimen, even when considerable inconvenience is involved, although the requirements emotionally lengthen the pregnancy time span for even the most cooperative patient.

THE IMPORTANCE OF A SUPPORT SYSTEM

Medical management support and family, peer, and employer attitudes are all influential in determining how a pregnant diabetic woman adapts to the diabetes and pregnancy regimen. The woman's motivation is heightened if the pregnancy is desired and planned by both partners and if she receives the necessary support from her mate or significant others. Good interfamilial relationships in existence before the pregnancy usually continue. However, any preexisting conflicts tend to become intensified as the regimen demands place additional strain on the relationship.

The health care professionals and family members should encourage the woman to accept help from others rather than acquiescing to the convenience of others. This "positive selfishness" is important for her own well-being and that of her baby, particularly for women who are used to managing everything themselves and find interdependency difficult to accept. Understanding and cooperation regarding medical appointments by employers can enhance a sense of well-being. Group discussions with other patients help develop camaraderie in sharing mutual experience.

The demanding diabetes and pregnancy regimen, with frequent tests and procedures, can create negative feelings in even the most cooperative patient. When recognized and allowed to be expressed, the frustration, fear, anger, and anxiety may be revealed and stress decreased. The health care professional should discuss with the patient what she can do to heighten her feelings of control over what is happening to her.

When a patient is under-insured or is without insurance coverage, a discussion about the cost of various tests and procedures should be initiated as the pregnancy progresses. The patient or her family may be reluctant to discuss this subject even though it may be of concern.

REFERENCES

1. Rao S, Lindow SW, Masson EA: Survey of pre-conception counselling. *Diabet Med* 19:615, 2002

2. Diabetes and Pregnancy Group: Knowledge about preconception care in French women with type 1 diabetes. *Diabetes Metab* 31:443–47, 2005

3. Hofmanova I: Pre-conception care and support for women with diabetes (Review). *Br J Nurs* 15:90–94, 2006

4. Chung JH, Voss KJ, Caughey AB, Wing DA, Henderson EJ, Major CA: Role of patient education level in predicting macrosomia among women with gestational diabetes mellitus. *J Perinatol* 26:328–32, 2006

5. Dunn SM, Turtle JR: The myth of the diabetic personality. *Diabetes Care* 4:640–46, 1981

6. Kahana R, Bibring D: Personality types in medical practice. In *Psychiatry and Medical Practice in a General Hospital*. New York, International University Press, 1964, p. 108–23

7. Barglow P, Hatcher R, Wolston J, Phelps R, Burns W, Depp R: Psychiatric risk factors in the pregnant diabetic patient. *Am J Obstet Gynecol* 140:46–52, 1981

8. Berezin N: *After a Loss in Pregnancy: Help for Families Affected by a Miscarriage, a Stillbirth or the Loss of a Newborn*. New York, Simon & Schuster, 1982

9. Law S: Patient cooperation: a determinant of perinatal outcome in the pregnant diabetic. *J Reprod Med* 24:197–200, 1980

10. Anderson RM: Patient empowerment and the traditional medical model: a case of irreconcilable differences? *Diabetes Care* 18:412–15, 1995

SUGGESTED READING

Bali C: Teaching intensive diabetes care in pregnancy: psychological aspects. *Diabetes Educ* 9:32s, 38s–40s, 47s, 1983

Barglow P, Hatcher R, Berndt D, Phelps R: Psychosocial childbearing stress and metabolic control in pregnant diabetics. *J Nerv Ment Dis* 173:615–20, 1985

Edelstein J, Linn MW: The influence of family in the control of diabetes. *Soc Sci Med* 21:541–44, 1985

Funnell MM, Anderson RM, Arnold MS, Barr PA, Donnelly MB, Johnson PD, Taylo-Moon D, White N: Empowerment: an idea whose time has come. *Diabetes Educ* 17:37–41, 1991

Hare E: The emotional experience of the pregnant diabetic woman: its impact on health care professionals. *Diabetes Educ* 9:35s–37s, 46s, 1989

Jovanovic-Peterson L: Do you really want this baby? *Diabetes Prof* Fall:16–18, 1989

Langer N, Langer O: Emotional adjustment and intensified treatment of gestational diabetes. *Obstet Gynecol* 84:3, 1994

Leff EW, Gagna MP, Jefferis SC: Type 1 diabetes and pregnancy...are hearing women's concerns? *Am J Nat Child Nurs* 16:83–187, 1991

Merkatz R, Budd K, Merkatz I: Psychological and social implications of scientific care for pregnant diabetic women. In *The Diabetic Pregnancy*. Merkatz R, Merkatz I, Adams PA, Eds. New York, Grune & Stratton, 1979, p. 93–101

Papatheodorou NH: The use of support groups in diabetes education. *Diabetes Educ* 7:40–42, 1981

Papatheodorou NH: Self-help support groups as an adjunct to diabetes education. *Diabetes Educ* 10:75–77, 1984

Papatheodorou NH: Pregnancy and diabetes: psychosocial perspectives. In *The Diabetic Pregnancy*. Nuwayhid B, Ed. New York, Elsevier, 1987, p. 137–67

Papatheodorou NH: Interactive communication in health-care delivery. *Diabetes Spectrum* 3:217–19, 254–55, 1990

Penha ML, Pichert JW, Mandeville LK: Diabetic mothers and pregnancy loss: implications for diabetes educators. *Diabetes Educ* 19:35–39, 1993

Quesado SF: Diabetes and pregnancy: use of an integrated team approach provides the necessary comprehensive care. *RI Med J* 72:129–32, 1989

Ruggiero L, Spirito A, Bond A, Coustan D, McGarvy ST: Impact of social support and stress on compliance in women with gestational diabetes. *Diabetes Care* 13:441–43, 1990

Ruggiero L, Spirito A, Bond A, Coustan D, McGarvy ST, Low RG: Self-reported compliance with diabetes self-management during pregnancy. *Int J Psychiatry Med* 23:195–207, 1993

St. James PJ, Younger MD, Hamilton BD, Waisbren SE: Unplanned pregnancies in young women with diabetes: an analysis of psychosocial factors. *Diabetes Care* 16:1572–78, 1993

Saling VR: Stress and intervention in gestational diabetes. *Diabetes Prof* Spring:28–35, 1990

Assessment of Glycemic Control

Highlights
Assessment of Glycemic Control

■ Hyperglycemia is the major cause of complications of diabetes and pregnancy.

■ Normoglycemia minimizes these complications.

■ Continued attention to blood glucose control is mandatory on the part of the woman and her health care team.

Assessment of Glycemic Control

Recent studies of intermittent capillary blood glucose and continuous interstitial glucose monitoring in normal women in their usual settings revealed a rather narrow range of glucose concentrations. Fasting plasma glucose concentrations decline in early normal pregnancy (1). There is a slight, gradual rise in mean and postprandial glucose values throughout the second and third trimesters of normal pregnancy. In nondiabetic pregnant women, the best reference ranges for capillary fasting, overnight, and premeal glucose calibrated to plasma levels are 50–99 mg/dl, with postmeal peak values 60–70 min after eating of 81–129 mg/dl (Table 11) (2,3).

SELF-MONITORING OF CAPILLARY BLOOD GLUCOSE

Self-monitoring of blood glucose (SMBG) is an integral part of the intensified treatment of diabetes that has dramatically improved pregnancy outcome over the last 25 years (4,5) and is necessary for individuals to achieve optimal glucose goals (6,7). Capillary blood glucose refers to the usual sample obtained by the patient; it is recognized that most glucose meters now calibrate capillary blood measurements to read as plasma glucose for comparability with reference laboratory measurements; hence, in this chapter, use of "SMBG" implies that fact. The amount of glucose per unit water mass is the same in whole blood and plasma. "Although red blood cells are essentially freely permeable to glucose (glucose is taken up by facilitated transport), the concentration of water in plasma (kg/l) is ~11% higher than that of whole blood. Therefore, glucose concentrations in plasma are ~11% higher than whole blood if the hematocrit is normal" (8). Because this is true for glucose values measured in venous or capillary blood (9–13), "it is crucial that people with diabetes know whether their monitor and strips provide whole blood or plasma results" (4). However, the recent National Academy of Clinical Biochemistry's guideline for management of diabetes adopted by the American Diabetes Association (5) suggests that the total error of meter use (user plus analytical) is often as much as the difference between whole blood and plasma glucose measurement, as noted by others (14,15). Variance of capillary glucose measurements compared with a reference plasma method seems to be greater the higher the glucose value (15). In studies of the accuracy of SMBG in the normo- to hyperglycemic range in diabetic pregnant women, usage of most home devices had a total error of <15% (16,17). In the hypoglycemic range, there may be a reduction in the accuracy of SMBG (18–20), perhaps because of alterations in subcutaneous

Table 11 Normal Glucose Concentrations (mg/dl) and A1C Levels During Third Trimester Pregnancy, Capillary Glucose and A1C Goals for Women with Preexisting Diabetes Before and During Early Pregnancy, and Optimal Goals During the Second and Third Trimesters

Group	Daily mean glucose	Fasting, premeal, nighttime	1-h post-prandial	A1C (%)
Normal pregnancy (mean and SD)				5.0 (0.4)**
Capillary glucose by meter* (2)	82.9 ± 5.8	69.3 ± 5.7	108.4 ± 6	
Continuous interstitial glucose (39)	83.7 ± 18	76.6 ± 11.5	105.3 ± 12	
Preexisting diabetes goals during the second and third trimesters	<110	60–99	100–129	<6.2

*Adjusted to be equivalent to plasma glucose values. **From refs. 48 and 49.

blood flow during hypoglycemia (21–23).

SMBG allows the patient to evaluate her individual response to therapy and assess whether glycemic targets are being achieved. Frequent sampling is optimal in pregnancy because of the increased potential for rapid-onset hypoglycemia in the absence of food or presence of exercise and the exacerbated hyperglycemic responses to food ingestion, psychological stress, and intercurrent illness related to gestational insulin resistance. Use of glucose meters with memory capacity is important for verification of the reliability of patient self-testing and recording (24). The accuracy of SMBG is instrument- and user-dependent (5), and it is important for health care providers to evaluate each patient's monitoring technique, both initially and at regular intervals thereafter. The patient should "use calibrators and controls on a regular basis to assure accuracy of results" (6). Optimal use of SMBG requires proper interpretation of the data, and many patients can be taught how to use the data to adjust food intake, exercise, or insulin therapy to achieve specific glycemic goals. Health care professionals regularly should evaluate the patients's ability to use data to guide therapy.

SITE OF SMBG

To provide less painful glucose self-testing, manufacturers developed products designed for use at alternate sites—usually the forearm or thigh (6). However, when glucose concentrations are rapidly rising or falling (e.g., postprandially, immediately after exercise, or with insulin-induced hypoglycemia), there is a lag time between the fingerstick capillary glucose concentration and the alternative site testing of the forearm and thigh (25–27). Therefore, use of alternative site testing systems in the dynamic state of pregnancy will give different results than fingerstick testing (6) and is not wise. Palm and fingertip capillary glucose values are similar at different time points (27,28), but these testing sites have not been compared in pregnancy.

TIMING OF SMBG

A randomized trial of premeal versus postprandial glucose testing as the guide for insulin therapy in pregnant women with rather severe GDM and fasting hyperglycemia reported lower frequencies of perinatal complications with the treatment strategy based on postmeal testing (29). A similar result was found in a randomized trial of premeal versus postprandial testing starting at 16 wk of gestation in type 1 diabetic patients (30). These trials support the previous observational studies in type 1 and type 2 diabetes that revealed postprandial glucose levels as the best predictor of fetal macrosomia (31–33). Because most pregnant patients with type 1 or type 2 diabetes will use short-acting insulin injections before meals to prevent postprandial hyperglycemia, premeal glucose testing is useful to allow temporary adjustments of insulin dose if the glucose level is low or elevated (34–37). Bedtime and overnight blood glucose testing is used as needed to detect hyper- or hypoglycemia at those time points to allow subsequent adjustment of snacks or insulin doses.

The protocols for the timing and frequency of self-monitored glucose concentrations should be designed to reflect the peak and the nadir of maternal glycemia. Previously when animal regular insulin was prescribed, and even with the advent of recombinant DNA technology that made available human regular insulin, the concern that the peak action of the regular insulin might cause hypoglycemic reactions 1.5–2.5 h after the injection led to usage of the 2-h postprandial time point. Because the available rapid-acting insulin analogs have peak effect at 45–70 min after injection, and because the concern is to prevent hyperglycemia-induced fetal complications, the evidence is mounting that 1-h postprandial testing may be better in most pregnancies complicated by diabetes. Studies with continuous interstitial glucose monitoring in diabetic pregnant women show the mean peak postprandial glucose to average 90 min after beginning the meal, with considerable variation from patient to patient (38) and high day-to-day variability (39). Teaching patients to test at 1 h after finishing the meal should approximate these peaks. Some pregnant patients may have delayed postprandial peak glucose excursions related to delayed gastric emptying (40). It is also recognized that meals with high fat content in pregnancy may prolong the postprandial glucose excursion. A study in which 68 women with GDM used SMBG at both 1 and 2 h postprandial for 1 wk after diagnosis revealed a greater proportion of abnormal values at 1 h after breakfast and equivalence after lunch, but a greater proportion of abnormal values at 2 h after dinner (41).

Continuous glucose monitoring (CGM) devices measure subcutaneous interstitial tissue glucose by an electrochemical method. Because interstitial fluid glucose levels are 20–50% lower than blood glucose levels (42), calibration with several capillary glucose levels per day corrects for this difference (43). Feasibility studies of older CGM systems in pregnancies of women with type 1 diabetes treated with multiple daily insulin injections revealed periods of both hyper- and hypoglycemia that were not detected by fingerstick testing or patient symptoms (38,43–46). However, interstitial glucose values failed to reflect symptomatic hypoglycemia confirmed by capillary glucose testing in 6.2% of all paired samples in a study of 15 pregnant women with type 1 diabetes (43), and reproducibility of glucose measurements in subjects wearing two sensors at the same time is not optimal (47–49). CGM devices provide real-time glucose data to patients and have alarms for both glucose values out of range and for rapidly changing glucose values. However, to make treatment decisions (such as calculating pre-meal insulin doses) patients are advised to use SMBG values. Prospective controlled trials are needed to determine if application of this expensive method to fine-tune glycemic control will improve perinatal outcome and maternal safety. Ancillary questions include which patients might benefit the most and at which stages of pregnancy.

OTHER MEASURES OF METABOLIC CONTROL

Glycated hemoglobin (GHb) is the general term used to describe a series of stable minor hemoglobin components formed slowly and nonenzymatically in direct proportion to the ambient glucose concentration (4). GHb values expressed as the percentage of total hemoglobin provide the best assessment of the degree of chronic glycemic control, reflecting the average blood glucose concentration during the preceding 6–12 wk because the lifespan of the red blood cells is shortened to <90 days in pregnancy (50). However, GHb can be misleading if patients balance frequent low and high blood glucose levels, since this indicator of average glucose would not reflect postprandial elevations, which could represent important pulses of high glucose in the fetus (51,52). Many GHb assays are available, but A1C has become the preferred standard for assessing glycemic control (4). When maternal glycemia is elevated and rapidly brought toward normal in pregnancy, A1C has been reported to show a significant decrease within 2 wk compared with the baseline elevation. Thus, the measurement of A1C every 2–4 wk confirms the SMBG measurements. Standardization of laboratory A1C measurements has been achieved by the vast majority of U.S. laboratories (6, 53, 54), since a variety of reference limits have been obtained with different high-performance liquid chromatography (HPLC) equipment (55). Manufacturers of A1C test methods can earn a certificate of traceability to the Diabetes Control and Complications Trial (DCCT) reference method (56) by passing rigorous testing criteria for precision and accuracy (4). One highly sensitive, precise, and accurate HPLC method yielded a reference range (2.5 and 97.5 percentiles) of 3.2–4.3 for 63 healthy pregnant women, compared with 3.4–4.9 in other adult women (55). Evaluation of DCCT-aligned ion exchange liquid chromatography assays revealed lower reference ranges for A1C in 493 and 100 healthy pregnant women of 4.1–5.9 and 4.5–5.7, respectively, compared with 4.7–6.3 in age-matched nonpregnant control women (57,58). The results were not affected by differences in body mass between groups. Trimester- and ethnic group–related differences in A1C in different stages of normal pregnancy are not of clinical significance (55,57,59).

Glycated serum protein assays correlate well with the A1C test (4). Although the measurement of fructosamine, an indirect measurement of glycosylated serum proteins (mostly albumin), theoretically should reflect the average blood glucose over the past week because of the rapid turnover rate of albumin (8 days in pregnancy), fructosamine has not proved to be useful in pregnancies complicated by diabetes. Because fructosamine assays are an indirect measurement of total glycosylated serum proteins, there is interference by reducing agents in the blood. If a pregnant woman has recently taken her prenatal vitamins, then the results of the fructosamine assay will vary based on her blood concentrations of vitamin C. Vitamin C concentrations in the blood alter the fructosamine assay more than small changes in glycemia. In addition, there is a diurnal variation in serum protein concentrations in the blood. Thus, the woman must have her fructosamine test at the same time for each determination or the variation in total serum proteins may be greater than the change in this measure of average blood glucose concentrations.

KETONURIA AND KETONEMIA

Ketone testing is important, since the presence of ketones can indicate impending diabetic ketoacidosis (DKA), which may develop quickly in pregnancy in type 1 diabetic women. Urine ketones should be measured periodically when the pregnant diabetic woman is ill or when any blood glucose value is >180 mg/dl. Outside pregnancy, 300 mg/dl is used, but a lower threshold is used in pregnancy because DKA can develop at lower levels of hyperglycemia in pregnant women with type 1 or type 2 diabetes (60). DKA is associated with a high mortality rate in the fetus (61). In addition, fasting ketonemia in poorly controlled pregnant diabetic women has been associated with decreased intelligence and fine motor skills in offspring (62). In early pregnancy, ketonuria sometimes occurs in women who are limiting their caloric intake because of nutritional recommendations or nausea and vomiting; however, it is unclear if starvation ketosis is associated with decreased intelligence in the offspring. Women with moderate to large ketonuria associated with hyperglycemia should alert their physician immediately for determination of ketonemia. Urine ketone tests are not reliable for the firm diagnosis of DKA, which is better made with blood ketone testing that quantifies β-hydroxybutyric acid (4). Home tests for β-hydroxybutyric acid are available, but they have not been evaluated systematically in pregnancy.

RECOMMENDATIONS

SMBG is a key component of diabetes therapy during pregnancy in both type 1 and type 2 diabetic patients and should be included in the management plan. Daily SMBG and testing both before and after meals will provide optimal results in pregnancy.

Fingerstick SMBG testing is best in pregnancy, since alternate site testing may not identify rapid changes in blood glucose concentrations characteristic of pregnant women with preexisting diabetes.

Instruct the patient in SMBG using meters with memory capacity, and routinely evaluate the patient's technique and ability to use data to adjust therapy. SMBG as used here implies current glucose meters that calibrate blood glucose readings to plasma glucose values. Ideally, provide the pregnant patient with the opportunity for daily telephone or electronic contact with the health care staff to discuss problems in management.

Postprandial capillary glucose measured 1 h after finishing the meal best approximates postmeal peak glucose measured continuously.

Because of individual differences in time to peak postprandial glucose level related to gastric emptying, content and time of meals, and possibly other factors, it may be optimal for each patient to determine her own peak postprandial glucose testing time after breakfast, lunch, and dinner.

Generally target fasting, overnight, and premeal plasma glucose values of 60–99 mg/dl, 1-h postmeal plasma glucose values of 100–129 mg/dl, and mean daily plasma glucose <100 mg/dl to achieve optimal pregnancy outcome.

SMBG targets must be tailored to individual patient characteristics, such as hypoglycemia unawareness.

Teach the patient to test capillary plasma glucose appropriately to prevent, identify, and treat hypoglycemia.

The use of continuous interstitial glucose monitoring needs more evaluation before it can be recommended for general use in pregnant diabetic women.

Teach the pregnant patient to perform urine ketone measurements at times of illness or when the blood glucose reaches 180 mg/dl. Positive values should be reported promptly to the health care professional.

Perform the A1C test at the initial visit during pregnancy and then monthly until target levels <6.2% in a DCCT-aligned assay are achieved; then every 2–4 mo should be sufficient.

REFERENCES

1. Mills JL, Jovanovic, L, Knopp R, Aarons J, Conley M, Park E, Lee YJ, Holmes L, Simpson JL, Metzger B: Physiological reduction in fasting blood glucose concentration in the first trimester of normal pregnancy: The Diabetes in Early Pregnancy Study. *Metabolism* 47:1140–44, 1998

2. Parretti E, Mecaci F, Papini M, Cioni R, Carignani L, Mignosa M, La Torre P, Mello G: Third-trimester maternal blood glucose levels from diurnal profiles in nondiabetic pregnancies: correlation with sonographic parameters of fetal growth. *Diabetes Care* 24:1319–23, 2001

3. Yogev Y, Ben-Haroush A, Chen R, Rosenn B, Hod M, Langer O: Diurnal glycemic profile in obese and normal weight nondiabetic pregnant women. *Am J Obstet Gynecol* 191:949–53, 2004

4. American Diabetes Association: Tests of glycemia in diabetes (Position Statement). *Diabetes Care* 27 (Suppl. 1):S91–93, 2004

5. Sacks DB, Bruns DE, Goldstein DE, Maclaren NK, McDonald JM, Parrott M: Guidelines and recommendations for laboratory analysis in the diagnosis and management of diabetes mellitus (Position Statement). *Diabetes Care* 25:750–86, 2002

6. Goldstein DE, Little RR, Lorenz RA, Malone JI, Nathan D, Peterson CM, Sacks DB: Tests of glycemia in diabetes (Technical Review). *Diabetes Care* 27:1761–73, 2004

7. The Diabetes Control and Complications Trial Research Group: Pregnancy outcomes in the Diabetes Control and Complications Trail. *American Journal of Obstetrics and Gynecology*, 174:1343–1353, 1996

8. Sacks DB, Bruns DE, Goldstein DE, Maclaren NK, McDonald JM, Parrott M: Guidelines and recommendations for laboratory analysis in the diagnosis and management of diabetes mellitus. *Clin Chem* 48:436–72, 2002

9. Chmielewski SA: Advances and strategies for glucose monitoring. *Am J Clin Pathol* 104 (Suppl. 1):S59–71, 1995

10. International Federation of Clinical Chemistry and Laboratory Medicine, Scientific Division Working Group on Selective Electrodes: IFCC recommendation on reporting results for blood glucose. *Clin Chim Acta* 307:205–09, 2001

11. Kuwa K, Nakayama T, Hoshino T, Tominaga M: Relationships of glucose concentrations in capillary whole blood, venous whole blood and venous plasma. *Clin Chim Acta* 307:187–92, 2001

12. Torjman MC, Jahn L, Joseph JI, Crothall K, Goldstein BJ: Accuracy of the HemoCue portable glucose analyzer in a large nonhomogeneous population. *Diabetes Technol Therapeut* 3:591–600, 2001

13. Buhling KJ, Henrich W, Kjos SL, Siebert G, Starr E, Dreweck C, Stein U, Dudenhausen JW: Comparison of point-of-care-testing glucose meters with standard laboratory measurement of the 50 g-glucose-challenge test (GCT) during pregnancy. *Clin Biochem* 36:333–37, 2003

14. Parkes JL, Slatin SL, Pardo S, Ginsberg BH: A new consensus error grid to evaluate the clinical significance of inaccuracies in the measurement of blood glucose. *Diabetes Care* 23:1143–48, 2000

15. Boehme P, Floriot M, Sirveaux M-A, Durain D, Ziegler O, Drouin P, Guerci B: Evolution of analytical performance in portable glucose meters in the last decade. *Diabetes Care* 26:1170–75, 2003

16. Moses R, Schier G, Mathews J, Davis W: The accuracy of home glucose meters for the glucose range anticipated in pregnancy. *Aust N Z J Obstet Gynecol* 37:282–86, 1997

17. Henry MJ, Major CA, Reinsch S: Accuracy of self-monitoring of blood glucose: impact on diabetes management decisions during pregnancy. *Diabetes Educ* 27:521–29, 2001

18. Moberg E, Lundblad S, Lins P-E, Adamson U: How accurate are home blood-glucose meters with special respect to the low glycemic range? *Diabetes Res Clin Pract* 19:239–43, 1993

19. Zenobi PD, Keller A, Jaeggi-Groisman SE, Glatz Y: Accuracy of devices for self-monitoring of blood glucose including hypoglycemic blood glucose levels. *Diabetes Care* 18:587–88, 1995

20. Trajanoski Z, Brunner GA, Gfrerer RJ, Wach P, Pieber TR: Accuracy of home blood glucose meters during hypoglycemia. *Diabetes Care* 19:1412–15, 1996

21. Hilsted J, Bonde-Petersen F, Madsbad S, Parving HH, Christensen NJ, Adelhoj B, Bigler D, Sjontoft E: Changes in plasma volume, in transcapillary escape rate of albumin and in subcutaneous blood flow during hypoglycemia in man. *Clin Sci* 69:273–77, 1985

22. Fernqvist-Forbes E, Linde B, Gunnarsson R: Insulin absorption and subcutaneous blood flow in normal subjects during hypoglycemia in man. *J Clin Endocrinol Metab* 67:619–23, 1988

23. Aman J, Berne C, Ewald U, Tuvemo T: Cutaneous blood flow during a hypoglycemic clamp in insulin-dependent diabetic patients and healthy subjects. *Clin Sci* 82:615–18, 1992

24. Langer O, Mazze RS: Diabetes in pregnancy: evaluating self-monitoring performance and glycemic control with memory-based reflectance meters. *Am J Obstet Gynecol* 155:635–37, 1986

25. Ellison JM, Stegman JM, Colner SL, Michael RH, Sharma MK, Ervin KR, Horwitz DL: Rapid changes in postprandial blood glucose produce concentration differences at finger, forearm, and thigh sampling sites. *Diabetes Care* 25:961–64, 2002

26. Jungheim K, Koschinsky T: Glucose monitoring in the arm: risky delays of hypoglycemia and hyperglycemia detection. *Diabetes Care* 25:956–60, 2002

27. Bina DM, Anderson RL, Johnson ML, Bergenstal RM, Kendall DM: Clinical impact of prandial state, exercise, and site preparation on the equivalence of alternative-site blood glucose testing. *Diabetes Care* 26:981–85, 2003

28. Meguro S, Funae O, Hosokawa K, Atsumi Y: Hypoglycemia detection rate differs among blood glucose monitoring sites. *Diabetes Care* 28:708–09, 2005

29. de Veciana M, Major CA, Morgan MA, Asrat T, Toohey JS, Lien JM, Evans AT: Postprandial versus preprandial blood glucose monitoring in women with gestational diabetes mellitus requiring insulin therapy. *N Engl J Med* 333:1237–41, 1995

30. Manderson JG, Patterson CC, Hadden DR, Traub AI, Ennis C, McCance DR: Preprandial versus postprandial blood glucose monitoring in type 1 diabetic pregnancy: a randomized controlled clinical trial. *Am J Obstet Gynecol* 189: 507–12, 2003

31. Jovanovic L, Peterson CM, Reed GF, Metzger BE, Mills JL, Knopp RH, Aarons JH: Maternal postprandial glucose levels and infant birth weight: the Diabetes in Early Pregnancy Study. The National Institute of Child Health and Human Development—Diabetes in Early Pregnancy Study. *Am J Obstet Gynecol* 164:103–111, 1991

32. Combs CA, Gunderson E, Kitzmiller JL, Gavin LA, Main EK: Relationship of fetal macrosomia to maternal postprandial glucose control during pregnancy. *Diabetes Care* 15:1251–57, 1992

33. Parretti E, Carignani L, Cioni R, Bartoli E, Borri P, La Torre P, Mecacci F, Martini E, Scarselli G, Mello G: Sonographic evaluation of fetal growth and body composition in women with different degrees of normal glucose metabolism. *Diabetes Care* 26:2741–48, 2003

34. Miller E, Hare JW, Cloherty JP, Dunn PJ, Gleason RE, Soeldner JS, Kitzmiller JL: Elevated maternal hemoglobin A1C in early pregnancy and major congenital anomalies in infants of diabetic mothers. *N Engl J Med* 304:1331–34, 1981

35. Jovanovic L, Druzin M, Peterson CM: Effect of euglycemia on the outcome of pregnancy in insulin-dependent diabetic women as compared with normal control subjects. *Am J Med* 71:921–27, 1981

36. Skyler JS, Skyler DL, Seigler DE, O'Sullivan MJ: Algorithms for adjustment of insulin dosage by patients who monitor blood glucose. *Diabetes Care* 4:311–18, 1981

37. Hirsch IB: Intensive treatment of type 1 diabetes. *Med Clin N Am* 82:689–719, 1998

38. Ben-Haroush A, Yogev Y, Chen R, Rosenn B, Hod M, Langer O: The postprandial glucose profile in the diabetic pregnancy. *Am J Obstet Gynecol* 191:576–81, 2004

39. Kerssen A, de Valk HW, Visser GHA: Day-to-day glucose variability during pregnancy in women with type 1 diabetes mellitus: glucose profiles measured with the continuous glucose monitoring system. *BJOG* 111:919–24, 2004

40. Stanley K, Magides A, Arnot M, Bruce C, Reilly C, McFee A, Fraser R: Delayed gastric emptying as a factor in delayed postprandial glycemic response in pregnancy. *Brit J Obstet Gynecol* 102:288–91, 1995

41. Sivan E, Weisz B, Homko CJ, Reece EA, Schiff E: One or two hours postprandial glucose measurements: are they the same? *Am J Obstet Gynecol* 185:604–07, 2001

42. Rebrin K, Steil GM, van Antwerp WP, Mastrototaro JJ: Subcutaneous glucose predicts plasma glucose independent of insulin: implications for continuous monitoring. *Am J Physiol* 277:E561–71, 1999

43. Kerssen A, de Valk HW, Visser GH: Do HbA1c levels and the self-monitoring of blood glucose levels adequately reflect glycemic control during pregnancy in women with type 1 diabetes mellitus? *Diabetologia* 49:25–8, 2006

44. Kerssen A, de valk HW, Visser GHA: The continuous glucose monitoring system during pregnancy of women with type 1 diabetes mellitus: accuracy assessment. *Diabetes Technol Ther* 6:645–51, 2004b

45. Yogev Y, Ben-Haroush A, Chen R, Kaplan B, Phillip M, Hod M: Continuous glucose monitoring for treatment adjustment in diabetic pregnancies: a pilot study. *Diabet Med* 20:558–62, 2003

46. Yogev Y, Chen R, Ben-Haroush A, Phillip M, Jovanovic L, Hod M: Continuous glucose monitoring for the evaluation of gravid women with type 1 diabetes mellitus. *Obstet Gynecol* 101:633–38, 2003

47. Metzger M, Leibowitz G, Wainstein J, Glaser B, Raz I: Reproducibility of glucose measurements using the glucose sensor. *Diabetes Care* 25:1185–91, 2002

48. Guerci B, Floriot M, Bohme P, Durain D, Benichou M, Jellimann S, Drouin P: Clinical performance of CGMS in type 1 diabetic patients treated by continuous subcutaneous glucose insulin infusion using insulin analogs. *Diabetes Care* 26:582–89, 2003

49. Larsen J, Ford T, Lyden E, Colling C, Mack-Shipman L, Lane J: What is

hypoglycemia in patients with well-controlled type 1 diabetes treated by subcutaneous insulin pump with use of the continuous glucose monitoring system? *Endocr Pract* 10:324–29, 2004

50. Lurie S, Danon D: Life span of erythrocytes in late pregnancy. *Obstet Gynecol* 80:123–26, 1992

51. Kerssen A, de Valk HW, Visser GH: Increased second trimester maternal glucose levels are related to extreme large-for-gestational age infants in women with type 1 diabetes mellitus. *Diabetes Care* 30:1069–74, 2007

52. Derr R, Garrett E, Stacy GA, Suadek CD: Is HbA1c affected by glycemic instability? *Diabetes Care* 26:2728–33, 2003

53. Sacks DB, ADA/EASD/IDF Working Group of the HbA1c Assay: Global harmonization of hemoglobin A1c. *Clin Chem* 51:681–3, 2005

54. Marshall SM, Barth JH: Standardization of HbA1c measurements: a consensus statement. *Diabet Med* 17:5–6, 2000

55. Parentoni LS, de Faria EC, Bartelega MJLF, Moda VMS, Facin ACC, Castilho LN: Glycated hemoglobin reference limits obtained by high performance liquid chromatography in adults and pregnant women. *Clin Chim Acta* 274:105–09, 1998

56. Rohlfing CL, Wiedmeyer HM, Little RR, England JD, Tennill A, Goldstein DE: Defining the relationship between plasma glucose and HbA1c: analysis of glucose profiles and HbA1c in the Diabetes Control and Complications Trial. *Diabetes Care* 25:275–78, 2002

57. O'Kane MJ, Lynch PLM, Moles KW, Magee SE: Determination of a Diabetes Control and Complications Trial-aligned HbA1c reference range in pregnancy. *Clin Chim Acta* 311:157–59, 2001

58. Nielsen LR, Ekbom P, Damm P, Glumer C, Frandsen MM, Jensen DM, Mathiesen ER: HbA1c levels are significantly lower in early and late pregnancy. *Diabetes Care* 27:1200–01, 2004

59. Hartland AJ, Smith JM, Clarke PMS, Webber J, Chowdhury T, Dunne F: Establishing trimester- and ethnic group-related reference ranges for fructosamine and HBA1c in non-diabetic pregnant women. *Ann Clin Biochem* 36:235–37, 1999

60. Whiteman VE, Homko CJ, Reece EA: Management of hypoglycemia and diabetic ketoacidosis in pregnancy. *Obstet Gynecol Clinics N Am* 23:87–107, 1996

61. Chauhan SP, Perry KG Jr: Management of diabetic ketoacidosis in the obstetric patient. *Obstet Gynecol Clinics N Am* 22:143–55, 1995

62. Rizzo T, Metzger BE, Burns WJ, Burns K: Correlations between antepartum maternal metabolism and child intelligence. *N Engl J Med* 325:911–16, 1991

Management of Morning Sickness

Highlights
Management of Morning Sickness

■ Patients suffering from morning sickness should eat six small meals each day, avoiding spicy and fatty foods and caffeine.

■ When nausea is a symptom of premeal hypoglycemia, options are to decrease the premeal insulin dose, shorten the insulin-meal interval, or have the patient take a portion of the insulin dose with a meal's carbohydrate to test tolerance before the rest of the insulin dose is taken.

■ If vomiting continues for >8 h, hospitalization for fluid replacement is advised. If intravenous therapy is required, blood glucose levels must remain in the normal range; glyccrol-based solutions are recommended because dextrose-based solutions carry with them a risk of hyperglycemia.

Management of Morning Sickness

Morning sickness—nausea or vomiting during pregnancy—is one of the most common symptoms of early pregnancy, affecting up to 70% of pregnant women (1,2). It is usually a tolerable annoyance for most women, but if the pregnant woman also has diabetes, the management of morning sickness requires special attention. Although it is termed morning sickness because it occurs most frequently on waking and lessens as the day continues, nausea and vomiting may occur at any time of day and even, on occasion, all day.

The cause of morning sickness is not completely understood, although relaxation of the smooth muscle of the stomach probably plays a role. The rapid rise of human chorionic gonadotropin (hCG) also may be implicated, however, because hyperemesis is associated with hydatidiform molar pregnancy, which manifests with hCG levels in the hundreds of thousands. The association between female sex of the fetus and hyperemesis gravidarum is not understood but is a known fact. In a retrospective study based on case notes of 166 women hospitalized for hyperemesis (3), female fetuses were significantly associated with severe starvation ketonemia and high urea. When vomiting resulted in severe dehydration during pregnancy, 85% of the fetuses were female. In recent studies assessing the utility of acupuncture (4) to eliminate the symptoms of hyperemsis, no significant effect was observed compared with the use of antiemetic medication. Because infants of mothers without diabetes with hyperemesis have a lower birth weight and are small for gestational age (5,6), in a diabetic pregnant woman, there must be additional caution taken to ensure strict glucose control and hydration to prevent first trimester complications associated with diabetes.

Typically, the symptoms begin 6 wk after the start of the last menstrual period and last 6–12 wk. The degree of nausea or vomiting a patient experiences and the sights or smells that trigger it can vary greatly from one pregnancy to another, although women who have had the problem before are somewhat more likely to experience it again. If it is a multiple gestation, symptoms are often more severe.

DIETARY REMEDIES

The treatment of morning sickness is seldom so successful that a woman will have complete relief. Time seems to be the only real cure. However, dietary changes can help minimize the discomfort and make the situation at least manageable (Table 12).

Usually, nausea is worse when the stomach is empty—hence the early-morning

Table 12 Tips for Controlling Nausea

- Eat dry crackers or toast before rising
- Eat small meals every 2.5–3 h
- Avoid caffeine
- Avoid fatty and spicy foods
- Drink fluids between meals, not with meals
- Take prenatal vitamins after dinner or at bedtime
- Always carry food

symptoms. For this reason, it is suggested that patients keep some starch, such as melba toast, rice cakes, saltines, or other low-fat crackers, at the bedside so they can eat if they become nauseated in the middle of the night or before getting out of bed in the morning. Eating a protein and carbohydrate snack at bedtime, such as cheese and crackers or half of a sandwich, will help prevent early-morning nausea. This snack also helps prevent the development of ketonuria, which may aggravate nausea.

To keep the stomach full, recommend to your patients that they eat six small meals per day. Generally, each meal should include food sources of carbohydrate, protein, and fat.

Table 13 illustrates an 1,800-calorie diet appropriate for a 5′4″ woman with a prepregnancy weight of 120 lb. It includes all the necessary nutrients and is designed to minimize nausea. Milk often aggravates nausea, so this diet limits milk consumption to 2 cups/day, but low-fat cheese or a calcium carbonate supplement can be added to meet calcium requirements. After the nausea has subsided, milk consumption should be increased to the recommended daily allowance for pregnancy of 4 cups. Fluids should be taken between meals rather than with meals (7).

Caffeine also may aggravate nausea, so advise a reduction in caffeine consumption. Fried, spicy, and fatty foods increase nausea. Peppers, chilies, and garlic are often culprits. Eating certain foods, or even simply smelling their aroma, can precipitate nausea, so advise patients to avoid these foods until the morning sickness has subsided. It may help if meals can be prepared by someone else. Taking prenatal vitamins after dinner or before bed may help decrease morning sickness.

INSULIN ADJUSTMENTS

Women with gestational diabetes who are treated with diet alone can usually manage their morning sickness with dietary remedies. The management of women with type 1 diabetes or insulin-treated type 2 diabetes who experience morning sickness provides a challenge for even the most skilled practitioners.

Nausea may be a symptom of hypoglycemia, and hypoglycemia often aggravates nausea. It is therefore essential to have your patients check their blood glucose often to avoid hypoglycemia.

It is also important that patients carry food at all times so that they can promptly

Table 13 1,800-Calorie Diet to Control Nausea

	Exchanges	Food Source
Before rising	1 Starch	6 crackers or 1 slice bread
Breakfast	1 Meat	1 oz low-fat cheese
	2 Starch	2 slices bread or 1 1/2 cups cereal
	1 Fat	1 tsp margarine
A.M. snack	1 Starch	3/4 cup cereal
	1 Milk	8 oz low-fat milk or plain yogurt
Lunch	2 Meat	1/2 cup tuna or 2 oz turkey or low-fat cheese
	1 Vegetable	1 cup salad or a medium tomato
	2 Starch	2 slices bread, 1 cup pasta, or 2/3 cup rice
	1 Fat	1 tsp mayonnaise or salad dressing
	1 Fruit	1/4 cantaloupe, 1 1/4 cup strawberries, or small nectarine
P.M. snack	1/2 Milk	4 oz low-fat milk
	1 Meat, 1 Starch	1/2 sandwich with 1 oz low-fat meat or cheese or 2 breadsticks with 1 oz low-fat cheese
Dinner	3 Meat	3 oz chicken or lean red meat, baked or broiled
	2 Vegetable	1 cup cooked vegetables (not potatoes, lima beans, peas, or other starch)
	2 Starch	2 slices bread, 1 cup pasta, or 2/3 cup rice
	1 Fat	1 tsp margarine
	1 Fruit	1 small peach
Bedtime snack	1/2 Milk	4 oz low-fat milk
	2 Starch	2 slices bread
	1 Meat	1 Tbsp peanut butter

treat any hypoglycemia or nausea. If nausea becomes severe enough to cause vomiting, women receiving insulin may need adjustments in the interval between their injection and meal.

When hypoglycemia is present and aggravating the nausea, the judicious use of subcutaneous glucagon may elevate the blood glucose sufficiently to alleviate the hypoglycemia-induced nausea and allow the patient to eat again. A dose of 0.15 mg s.c. glucagon raises the blood glucose ~30 mg/dl (~2 mmol/l) (7). Glucagon is also useful if the patient has taken her premeal dose of short-acting insulin and then vomited the meal. In this case, a dose of 0.15 mg s.c. glucagon should also be given but may need to be repeated every 1–2 h until the peak short-acting insulin action has declined.

There are several approaches for decreasing premeal hypoglycemia and nausea:

- Take rapid-acting insulin after eating once blood glucose levels begin to rise.
- Have patients take a portion of the insulin with a small part of the meal's carbohydrate to see how well the food is tolerated before taking the remainder of the insulin and the meal.

If a patient cannot tolerate food and has vomited after a meal, recommend that she initially substitute tomato juice for the meal (12 oz juice has 15 g carbohydrate), because fluids may be more easily tolerated. Once the vomiting has subsided, she can eat the remainder of the meal. Advise patients who have vomited to check their blood glucose and urine ketone levels frequently.

MEDICAL MANAGEMENT

If vomiting during pregnancy is not controlled by dietary remedies and becomes severe, many practitioners advise hospitalization to prevent dehydration, electrolyte disturbances, and weight loss. It is best to recommend hospitalization if vomiting continues for 8 h, the patient has persistent hypoglycemia, or the patient has developed significant ketonuria. Treatment usually consists of intravenous fluids, potassium replacement, and close monitoring of blood glucose, urine ketones, and weight. Antiemetic medications also may be needed until the cycle of vomiting has been stopped.

Nausea and vomiting during pregnancy that is severe enough to cause dehydration is known as hyperemesis gravidarum. Hyperemesis occurs in 0.3–0.4% of pregnant women. Although this condition represents a severe complication of pregnancy without type 1 diabetes (8–11), any woman with hyperemesis and diabetes generally requires initial hospitalization. If the community has a nutritional support team that can manage home parenteral nutrition, it may be possible to manage the patient at home. At all costs, the mother's blood glucose levels should be kept in the normal range despite the intravenous therapy. Because of this, glycerol-based solutions, rather than dextrose-based solutions, are recommended.

There are no medications available that are indicated specifically for the treatment of nausea and vomiting during pregnancy. Some physicians prescribe antiemetic medications for severe nausea and vomiting. The dangers of dehydration and electrolyte imbalance must be weighed against any risks associated with antiemetics.

The best reassurance for patients is that the "tincture of time" is the best medicine. For most women, symptoms are generally lessened once they have eaten and are markedly diminished by the end of the fourth month. Women experiencing morning sickness are statistically less likely to experience a spontaneous loss or preterm birth (10,11). This can be especially reassuring information for women with diabetes.

REFERENCES

1. Cunningham FG, MacDonald PC, Gant NS (Eds.): Management of normal pregnancy. In *Williams Obstetrics*. 18th ed. Norwalk, CT, Appleton & Lange, 1989, p. 270–71

2. Vellacott ID, Cooke EJ, James CE: Nausea and vomiting in early pregnancy. *Int J Gynaecol Obstet* 27:57–62, 1988

3. Tan PC, Jacob R, Quek KF, Omar SZ: The fetal sex ratio and metabolic, biochemical, haematological and clinical indicators of severity of hyperemesis gravidarum. *BJOG* 113:733–37, 2006

4. Heazell A, Thorneycroft J, Walton V, Etherington I: Acupressure for the in-patient treatment of nausea and vomiting in early pregnancy: a randomized control trial. *Am J Obstet Gynecol* 194:815–20, 2006

5. Dodds L, Fell DB, Joseph KS, Allen VM, Butler B: Outcomes of pregnancies complicated by hyperemesis gravidarum. *Obstet Gynecol* 107:285–92, 2006

6. Bailit JL: Hyperemesis gravidarium: epidemiologic findings from a large cohort. *Am J Obstet Gynecol* 193:811–84, 2005

7. Jovanovic L, Druzin M, Peterson CM: *Protocols for Managing Type 1 Diabetic Women*. Indianapolis, IN, Boehringer Mannheim, 1986

8. Jornsay DL: Managing morning sickness. *Diabetes Self-Management* 10:10–12, 1990

9. Gross S, Librach C, Cecutti A: Maternal weight loss associated with hyperemesis gravidarum: a predictor of fetal outcome. *Am J Obstet Gynecol* 160:906–09, 1989

10. Weigel MM, Weigel RM: Nausea and vomiting of early pregnancy and pregnancy outcome: an epidemiological study. *Br J Obstet Gynaecol* 96:1304–11, 1989

11. Weigel RM, Weigel MM: Nausea and vomiting of early pregnancy and pregnancy outcome: a meta-analytical review. *Br J Obstet Gynaecol* 96:1312–18, 1989

Nutritional Management During Pregnancy in Preexisting Diabetes

Highlights
Nutritional Management
During Pregnancy in
Preexisting Diabetes

■ Patient responsibility is the cornerstone of nutritional management for women with diabetes.

■ The nutrient needs of pregnant women with diabetes are based on the Institute of Medicine's 2006 Dietary Reference Intakes for Women, summarized in Table 14.

■ Dietary assessment and the development of a meal plan should be conducted individually by a registered dietitian.

■ Calorie levels and weight gain recommendations depend on the woman's prepregnancy weight.

■ Nutritional management of postpartum women with diabetes is addressed—specifically the requirements during lactation.

Nutritional Management During Pregnancy in Preexisting Diabetes

Adequate nutrition is one of the most important influences on the health of pregnant women and their infants. Suboptimal maternal nutritional status can compromise pregnancy outcome and increase the prevalence of low birth weight. A decreased prevalence of preeclampsia, prematurity, and neonatal morbidity and mortality has been reported when nutritional services and dietary supplements are given to pregnant women at nutritional risk. In pregnant women with diabetes, an adequate diet, appropriate weight gain, and maintenance of normoglycemia are critical for maintaining maternal body tissues and for optimal fetal growth and development.

PATIENT RESPONSIBILITY

The pregnant woman with diabetes should not be a passive recipient of health care, but should be the primary active member of the treatment team. She must understand that what she eats affects the health of her developing baby. The patient is in charge; she must take control of her diet, check her blood glucose, and keep records. Patients are usually highly motivated once they understand the importance of well-controlled diabetes to the health of their unborn baby.

NUTRIENT NEEDS OF PREGNANCY

The nutrient needs during pregnancy were revised by the Institute of Medicine in 2006. Table 14 shows the dietary reference intakes for nonpregnant, pregnant, and lactating women. Some nutrients of particular concern during pregnancy are briefly discussed below.

PROTEIN

Additional protein is required during pregnancy for the expansion of maternal plasma volume and amniotic fluid and to support the growth of placental, fetal, and maternal tissue. The recommended dietary allowance (RDA) for protein in the nonpregnant woman is 0.8 g/kg/day. During the second and third trimester, the requirement increases to 1.1 g/kg/day or ~25 g/day.

Table 14. Dietary Reference Intakes for Women[a,b]

Nutrient	Adult woman	Pregnancy	Lactation (0–6 mo)
Energy (kcal)	2,403	2,743[c], 2,855[d]	2,698
Protein (g/kg/d)	0.8	1.1	1.1
Carbohydrate (g/d)	130	175	210
Total fiber (g/d)	25	28	29
Linoleic acid (g/d)	12	13	13
α-Linolenic acid (g/d)	12	13	13
Vitamin A (µg RAE[e])	700	770	1,300
Vitamin D (µg)	5	5	5
Vitamin E (mg α-tocopherol)	15	15	19
Vitamin K (µg)	90	90	90
Vitamin C (mg)	75	85	120
Thiamin (mg)	1.1	1.4	1.4
Riboflavin (mg)	1.1	1.4	1.6
Vitamin B-6 (mg)	1.3	1.9	2.0
Niacin (mg NE[f])	14	18	17
Folate (µg dietary folate equivalents)	400	600	500
Vitamin B-12 (µg)	2.4	2.6	2.8
Pantothenic acid (mg)	5	6	7
Biotin (µg)	30	30	35
Choline (mg)	425	450	550
Calcium (mg)	1,000	1,000	1,000
Phosphorus (mg)	700	700	700
Magnesium (mg)	320	350	310
Iron (mg)	8	27	9
Zinc (mg)	8	11	12
Iodine (µg)	150	220	290
Selenium (µg)	55	60	70
Fluoride (mg)	3	3	3
Manganese (mg)	1.8	2.0	2.6
Molybdenum (µg)	45	50	50
Chromium (µg)	25	30	45
Copper (µg)	900	1,000	1,300
Sodium (mg)	2,300	2,300	2,300
Potassium (mg)	4,700	4,700	5,100

[a] Data from *Institute of Medicine, Dietary Reference Intakes: The Essential Guide to Nutrient Requirements,* Washington, DC, National Academies Press, 2006.

[b] Values are Recommended Dietary Allowances except energy (Estimated Energy Requirement) and total fiber, linoleic acid, α-linolenic acid, vitamin D, vitamin K, pantothenic acid, biotin, choline, calcium, manganese, chromium, sodium, and potassium (Adequate intakes).

[c] Second trimester for women age 19 to 50 years.

[d] Third trimester for women 19 to 50 years.

[e] RAE = retinal activity equivalents.

[f] NE = niacin equivalents

CALORIES

Pregnancy imposes additional energy needs because of added maternal tissues and growth of the fetus and placenta. Adequate maternal weight gain, including some maternal fat storage, is needed to ensure that the size of the newborn is optimal for survival. Storage of energy is included as part of the energy requirement of pregnancy. Nonpregnant American women of average height and stable weight ingest ~2,400 kcal/day (1). An additional 340 kcal/day is recommended during the second trimester, and 452 kcal/day is recommended during the third trimester. Energy requirements are determined individually for pregnant women with type 1, or insulin-requiring, diabetes and are discussed below.

DIETARY FAT

There are no RDAs for dietary fat intake during pregnancy. The recommended range for fat is 20–35% of total calories. Less than 10% of calories should be derived from saturated fats and less than 10% from polyunsaturated fats, with the remainder from monounsaturated fats. The adequate intake for essential fatty acids in pregnancy is 13 g/day of omega-6 and 1.4 g/day of omega-3 (1). Docosahexaenoic acid, a polyunsaturated fatty acid necessary for fetal development, is found mainly in cold water fish such as salmon. Pregnant women are advised not to consume certain large predatory fish, such as shark, tilefish, king mackerel, and swordfish, because of high mercury levels.

FOLATE

Folate functions as a coenzyme in the transfer of single carbon units from one compound to another. A folate deficiency during early gestation is associated with impaired cellular growth and replication resulting in fetal malformations, spontaneous abortions, preterm delivery, and low birth weight (2). As a result of the evidence of folate's role in the prevention of neural tube defects, the U.S. Public Health Service recommends that all women in their childbearing years consume 400 µg/day folic acid. Women with a previous neural tube defect pregnancy are advised to take 4 mg/day folate. The Institute of Medicine recommends an increase to 600 µg/day during pregnancy (1). There has been a decrease in neural tube defects since the U.S. Public Health Service recommendations and a greater reduction after the mandatory fortification of grain products with folic acid in 1998 (3,4). Health care providers must encourage an adequate daily intake of folic acid through the consumption of fortified foods and/or supplements.

CALCIUM AND VITAMIN D

Calcium absorption increases in pregnancy. As a result, the RDA for calcium in pregnancy is 1,000 mg/day, the same as for nonpregnant individuals (1).

Vitamin D is necessary to maintain positive calcium homeostasis in pregnancy. A deficiency in vitamin D may lead to inadequate calcium deposition in the fetal bone. The adequate intake for vitamin D in pregnancy is 5 µg/day (1). Sunlight and vitamin-fortified milk are two of the best sources of vitamin D. Recent studies have shown that dark-skinned and covered women are at increased risk of vitamin D deficiency if they had limited exposure to sunlight and did not consume fortified milk. Low blood levels of 25-hydroxycholecalciferol were observed and their infants were at risk of developing rickets and hypocalcemia (5). Vegans may need to supplement their diets with vitamin D.

IRON

The RDA for iron is 27 mg/day throughout pregnancy (6). Although iron absorption increases during pregnancy, extra iron is required for fetal erythropoesis and an increase in maternal red cell mass. Unless there is evidence of an iron deficiency in the first trimester, iron supplementation should be initiated in the second trimester (2). The Institute of Medicine recommends a low-dose supplementation of 30 mg/day of elemental iron, usually found in most prenatal vitamin/mineral supplements. Women with anemia may need 60 mg/day iron supplementation until the anemia is resolved.

Iron deficiency in pregnancy increases risk of low birth weight and may increase the risks of preterm delivery and perinatal mortality (7).

ZINC

Zinc is an important component in the metabolism of nucleic acids. The RDA for zinc in pregnancy is 11–13 g/day, an increase of 3 g over nonpregnant requirements (6). Zinc deficiency in pregnancy is associated with pregnancy-induced hypertension, congenital malformations, intrauterine growth retardation, and premature birth. Alcohol, tobacco, and iron supplementation may interfere with zinc absorption. Zinc supplementation is recommended if >30 mg/day of elemental iron is prescribed.

CHROMIUM

The role of chromium in diabetes management has been extensively studied. Chromium is believed to improve glucose tolerance, increase insulin sensitivity, and decrease insulin resistance (8). The RDA for chromium in pregnancy is 30 µg/day, preferably from food sources (6).

ASSESSING DIET AND EATING HABITS

A dietary assessment should be conducted to determine whether the woman's intake of essential nutrients is adequate and whether she is eating excessive amounts of fat, sugar, salt, or artificial sweeteners. It also allows for the identification of food avoidances, intolerances, or allergies that may limit food or nutrient intake.

An inadequate intake of essential nutrients predisposes a woman to deficiencies that can affect the course and outcome of her pregnancy. After smoking, poor gestational nutrition is the second most important risk factor for intrauterine growth retardation and low birth weight.

A prenatal nutrition questionnaire helps the practitioner to identify pregnancy-related problems affecting appetite and nutritional status (e.g., nausea, vomiting, heartburn, diarrhea, constipation). A patient's food preferences, aversions, cravings, and special diets should be identified and used to develop the meal plan with the patient. The patient should be referred to a registered dietitian for development of an individualized meal plan and medical nutrition therapy to meet weight and glycemic goals.

To assess the nutrient adequacy of the patient's diet, food records must be analyzed, along with blood glucose self-monitoring records. The timing of meals and snacks, amounts of foods, and preparation methods must be determined. In addition, the dietitian needs to look at the patient's blood glucose values and insulin schedule to determine whether the diet meets her nutritional requirements while allowing her to achieve or maintain normoglycemia. The dietitian should assess the diet for protein, carbohydrate, fat, calories, and major nutrients and compare it to the dietary reference intakes to assess nutrient adequacy. Recommendations for caloric level and ideal weight gain ranges should be made individually and are discussed below.

VITAMIN/MINERAL SUPPLEMENTATION

If the woman is motivated and knowledgeable and has enough income to follow a nutritionally adequate diet, iron and folate are the only nutrients that need to be routinely prescribed during pregnancy. However, carefully selected vitamin and mineral supplements are recommended for women at nutritional risk. A multivitamin/mineral preparation containing iron, zinc, copper, calcium, vitamin B6, folate, vitamin C, and vitamin D is recommended for women with inadequate dietary intakes or special problems. Supplementation cannot compensate for poor food habits. To be truly well nourished, pregnant women should be encouraged to eat an adequate quantity of a wide variety of nutritious foods (7).

DETERMINING CALORIE LEVEL

The appropriate calorie level of the diet depends on the patient's pregravid weight. Adequate calories are needed for optimal weight gain and to prevent starvation ketosis during the second and third trimesters of pregnancy (Table 15).

Table 15 Recommended Daily Caloric Intake

Pregnancy BMI Category	kcal/kg/day	kcal/lb/day
Low (BMI <18.5 kg/m²)	36–40	16.3–18.2
Normal (BMI 18.5–24.9 kg/m²)	30	13.6
High (BMI 25–29.9 kg/m²)	24	10.9
Obese (BMI >29.9 kg/m²)	12	5.4

Table 16. Body Mass Index Table

BMI	Normal						Overweight					Obese										Extreme Obesity														
	19	20	21	22	23	24	25	26	27	28	29	30	31	32	33	34	35	36	37	38	39	40	41	42	43	44	45	46	47	48	49	50	51	52	53	54
Height (inches)												**Body Weight (pounds)**																								
58	91	96	100	105	110	115	119	124	129	134	138	143	148	153	158	162	167	172	177	181	186	191	196	201	205	210	215	220	224	229	234	239	244	248	253	258
59	94	99	104	109	114	119	124	128	133	138	143	148	153	158	163	168	173	178	183	188	193	198	203	208	212	217	222	227	232	237	242	247	252	257	262	267
60	97	102	107	112	118	123	128	133	138	143	148	153	158	163	168	174	179	184	189	194	199	204	209	215	220	225	230	235	240	245	250	255	261	266	271	276
61	100	106	111	116	122	127	132	137	143	148	153	158	164	169	174	180	185	190	195	201	206	211	217	222	227	232	238	243	248	254	259	264	269	275	280	285
62	104	109	115	120	126	131	136	142	147	153	158	164	169	175	180	186	191	196	202	207	213	218	224	229	235	240	246	251	256	262	267	273	278	284	289	295
63	107	113	118	124	130	135	141	146	152	158	163	169	175	180	186	191	197	203	208	214	220	225	231	237	242	248	254	259	265	270	278	282	287	293	299	304
64	110	116	122	128	134	140	145	151	157	163	169	174	180	186	192	197	204	209	215	221	227	232	238	244	250	256	262	267	273	279	285	291	296	302	308	314
65	114	120	126	132	138	144	150	156	162	168	174	180	186	192	198	204	210	216	222	228	234	240	246	252	258	264	270	276	282	288	294	300	306	312	318	324
66	118	124	130	136	142	148	155	161	167	173	179	186	192	198	204	210	216	223	229	235	241	247	253	260	266	272	278	284	291	297	303	309	315	322	328	334
67	121	127	134	140	146	153	159	166	172	178	185	191	198	204	211	217	223	230	236	242	249	255	261	268	274	280	287	293	299	306	312	319	325	331	338	344
68	125	131	138	144	151	158	164	171	177	184	190	197	203	210	216	223	230	236	243	249	256	262	269	276	282	289	295	302	308	315	322	328	335	341	348	354
69	128	135	142	149	155	162	169	176	182	189	196	203	209	216	223	230	236	243	250	257	263	270	277	284	291	297	304	311	318	324	331	338	345	351	358	365
70	132	139	146	153	160	167	174	181	188	195	202	209	216	222	229	236	243	250	257	264	271	278	285	292	299	306	313	320	327	334	341	348	355	362	369	376
71	136	143	150	157	165	172	179	186	193	200	208	215	222	229	236	243	250	257	265	272	279	286	293	301	308	315	322	329	338	343	351	358	365	372	379	386
72	140	147	154	162	169	177	184	191	199	206	213	221	228	235	242	250	258	265	272	279	287	294	302	309	316	324	331	338	346	353	361	368	375	383	390	397
73	144	151	159	166	174	182	189	197	204	212	219	227	235	242	250	257	265	272	280	288	295	302	310	318	325	333	340	348	355	363	371	378	386	393	401	408
74	148	155	163	171	179	186	194	202	210	218	225	233	241	249	256	264	272	280	287	295	303	311	319	326	334	342	350	358	365	373	381	389	396	404	412	420
75	152	160	168	176	184	192	200	208	216	224	232	240	248	256	264	272	279	287	295	303	311	319	327	335	343	351	359	367	375	383	391	399	407	415	423	431
76	156	164	172	180	189	197	205	213	221	230	238	246	254	263	271	279	287	295	304	312	320	328	336	344	353	361	369	377	385	394	402	410	418	426	435	443

Adapted from Clinical Guidelines on the Identification, Evaluation, and Treatment of Overweight and Obesity in Adults: The Evidence Report.

WEIGHT GAIN

In women entering pregnancy within the normal BMI range (19.8–26 kg/m²), weight gains between 25 and 35 lb are associated with the most optimal outcomes. Women who gain amounts in this range have the lowest incidence of obstetric complications and premature births (2).

Women who are underweight (BMI <19.8 kg/m²) before conception should gain 28–40 lb to increase their depleted nutrient and energy stores and improve the chance of delivering an infant of desirable weight. Overweight women (BMI >26–29 kg/m²) do not need to gain as much weight because of their existing adipose tissue. Appropriate weight gain for these women is ≤15 lbs.

For women with diabetes, as long as the woman is consuming a nutritionally adequate diet, blood glucose levels are in the acceptable range, and other maternal/fetal parameters are normal, weight gain is monitored individually. Table 16 is a reference for determining BMI. Table 17 summarizes recommended weight gain ranges (2,9).

These are general guidelines. Women who have already met or exceeded these ranges before delivery should not have their weight gain severely restricted. Any indicated weight reduction should await the postpartum period.

The optimal pattern of weight gain is a very gradual process. During the first trimester, the usual gain is 2–5 lb. The weight is primarily due to increased blood volume and the growth of the uterus. During the second and third trimesters, 0.5–1 lb/week is a desirable weight gain range. In the second trimester, weight gain is due to major changes in the mother's body to support the pregnancy. The third trimester represents maximal growth of the baby and placenta.

MEAL PLANNING: DISTRIBUTING CALORIES AND CARBOHYDRATES

The recommended calorie distribution is as follows: 40% carbohydrate, 20% protein, and 30–40% fat.

Table 17. Weight Gain Recommendations During Pregnancy

Prepregnancy BMI (kg/m²)	Prepregnancy Weight Classification or Pregnancy Type	Recommended Weight Gain (pounds)
<19.8	Underweight or low	28–40
19.8–26	Normal or Ideal	25–35
>26–29	Overweight	15–25
>29	Obese	≥15
	Twin pregnancy	25–35
	Triplet pregnancy	≥50

Reprinted with permission. Sources (2,9).

CARBOHYDRATE

The amount, type, and distribution of carbohydrates should be based on blood glucose, weight gain, physical activity, and insulin therapy (10). During pregnancy, the preferred form of carbohydrate is that found in starches, legumes, and vegetables. These foods are often more nutrient dense, and their inclusion in the diet improves its nutritional adequacy. Initially, processed foods high in sugars are discouraged; many are lacking in essential nutrients and may have an adverse effect on postprandial blood glucose levels. The types of carbohydrate included in the diet must be individualized: if normoglycemia is achieved and maintained, more sugars may be included in the meal plan.

Postprandial blood glucose level depends on the carbohydrate content of the meal (11). Because postprandial blood glucose plays a major role in the development of neonatal macrosomia (12), a "euglycemic diet" designed to blunt postprandial hyperglycemia is effective. American Diabetes Association nutrition recommendations state that "the percentage of calories from carbohydrate will also vary and is individualized based on the patient's eating habits and glucose and lipid goals" (13). As a starting point, many practitioners find that a carbohydrate level of no more than 40% of calories is necessary to maintain euglycemia (14,15).

When rapid-acting insulin is given before meals, its action is optimized by minimizing the carbohydrate content of the meal. If a 55% carbohydrate diet is prescribed, then large doses of short-acting insulin are needed to maintain postprandial blood glucose level in the normal range. However, such large insulin doses result in between-meal hypoglycemia.

The Sweet Success California Diabetes and Pregnancy Program recommends the meal plan for diabetes in pregnancy consist of 40–45% of calories from carbohydrate, with a minimum of 175 g CHO/day (16). Women who are insulin resistant may need to have the percentage of carbohydrate in the diet reduced to 33% of calories (11).

Many practitioners start a patient on a diet of 40% of calories as carbohydrate. This is then liberalized if the patient successfully masters matching dietary carbohydrate to insulin. The postprandial glycemic rise is primarily affected by dietary carbohydrate, so patients should learn how to measure the amount of carbohydrates in foods and to adjust insulin to prevent hyper- or hypoglycemia.

FINE-TUNING: MATCHING CARBOHYDRATE TO INSULIN

Because the amount of carbohydrate in the diet directly affects the glycemic response, the amount of short-acting insulin a patient takes may be matched with the planned carbohydrate content of the meal. A fixed mixture of insulins is not recommended because it is difficult to manipulate for adjustments in meal plans.

A scale of rapid-acting insulin is used, based on the patient's preprandial blood glucose. When blood glucose is in the normal range, this formula is an example for matching dietary carbohydrate to short-acting insulin:

- 1.5 U short-acting insulin per 10 g carbohydrate at breakfast
- 1 U short-acting insulin per 10 g carbohydrate at lunch and dinner

The body is more insulin resistant in the morning; therefore, more insulin is required before breakfast. Insulin needs to be adjusted upward if preprandial blood glucose is elevated or downward if preprandial blood glucose is lower than normal (Table 18; see also page 94).

DEVELOPING THE MEAL PLAN

Food, especially dietary carbohydrate, must be balanced with insulin to avoid insulin reactions and provide for a sustained release of glucose. The timing and number of meals must be individually adjusted for lifestyle and physical activity.

In developing the meal plan with the patient, the food exchange system or carbohydrate counting may be used for making food selections. The meal plan must be individually tailored, based on nutrition/dietary assessment. Food models, measuring cups and spoons, and common household cups, glasses, and bowls are helpful props to use when teaching appropriate serving sizes. Key nutrients and their role in fetal growth and development should be briefly explained at this time.

Once the meal pattern has been developed, the patient and dietitian should develop a sample menu. This exercise helps the patient understand the exchange system or carbohydrate counting and helps the dietitian evaluate the patient's working knowledge of the prescribed diet. One example of the calorie distribution of meals and snacks is:

- 10% of calories at breakfast
- 20–30% of calories at lunch
- 30–40% of calories at dinner
- 30% of calories as snacks as needed

A sample diet plan for a normal-weight 60-kg (132-lb) pregnant woman is shown in Table 19.

If our sample woman was taking short-acting insulin before breakfast and dinner and her blood glucose levels were in the normal range before these meals, she would take 2 U insulin before breakfast and 7 U insulin before dinner:

- Breakfast of 15 g carbohydrate (1.5 U/10 g) = 2 U insulin
- Dinner of 67 g carbohydrate (1 U/10 g) = 7 U insulin

This system allows the patient dietary flexibility and control.

Table 18 Sample Sliding Scale for Matching Insulin to Food Intake

Blood Glucose	Insulin
<70 mg/dl (<3.8 mmol/l)	$X - 2$ U regular
70–100 mg/dl (3.8–5.5 mmol/l)	X
100–140 mg/dl (5.5–7.8 mmol/l)	$X + 2$ U regular
>140 mg/dl (>7.8 mmol/l)	$X + 4$ U regular

X = 1.5 U regular short-acting insulin for every 10 g carbohydrate eaten at breakfast or 1 U regular insulin for every 10 g carbohydrate at lunch or dinner.

Table 19 Sample 1,800-kcal Menu With 40% (180 g) Carbohydrate for 60-kg Pregnant Woman

Meal	Carbohydrate (g)	kcal (%)
Breakfast		
1 egg	0	100
1 slice whole-wheat toast	15	80
1 caffeine-free tea or coffee	0	0
		180 (10)
Snack		
1 medium apple	15	60
1 oz cheese	0	100
		160 (10)
Lunch		
2 slices whole-wheat bread	30	160
2 oz water-packed tuna	0	110
Tossed green salad	10	50
2 tsp mayonnaise	0	90
		410 (20)
Snack		
6 whole-wheat crackers	15	80
1 Tbsp sugar-free peanut butter	0	100
Caffeine-free iced tea		0
		180 (10)
Dinner		
4 oz lean meat, fish, or poultry	0	220
1 small baked potato	15	80
1/2 cup steamed broccoli and		
1/2 cup carrots	12	53
1 piece fruit	15	60
8 oz fat-free milk	12	100
1 whole-wheat roll	15	80
3 tsp margarine	0	135
		728 (40)
Snack		
8 oz fat-free milk	12	90
1/2 cup high-fiber cereal	15	80
		170 (10)
Total	181	1,828 (100)

FIBER

Foods high in soluble fibers, such as beans, fruit, and oat bran, help control diabetes by preventing dramatic swings in blood glucose levels. Soluble fibers form gels that delay the absorption of nutrients from the intestine. This slowed absorption allows for a more gradual influx of glucose into the blood, creating less of an insulin demand.

Insoluble fiber (such as wheat bran) cannot be digested and speeds the movement of food through the gastrointestinal tract. This type of fiber increases fecal bulk and contributes to regularity. In general, high-fiber foods are preferable for pregnant women with diabetes because they are nutrient dense.

PROTEIN

Lean protein foods should be encouraged, such as poultry without skin, boiled beans, and lean cuts of meat. Because of the recent concerns about the mercury content of fish, pregnant women are advised not to consume certain large predatory fish (shark, tilefish, king mackerel, swordfish).

FAT

According to the American Diabetes Association nutrition guidelines, "the distribution of calories from fat and carbohydrate can vary and be individualized based on the nutritional assessment and treatment goals" (13). To achieve normoglycemia, dietary fat may be liberalized (up to 40% of daily calories) (15). If the carbohydrate content of the diet is decreased to maintain normoglycemia, additional calories can come from fat. (Protein calories may also be increased, but this makes the diet more expensive.) Less than one-third of the fat calories each day should be from saturated fat and less than one-third from polyunsaturated fat; the balance should come from monounsaturated fats. The dietary guidelines in Table 20 should be given to overweight women or women whose gestational weight gain is excessive to improve the nutritional adequacy of the diet.

Table 20 Dietary Guidelines for Reducing Fat Intake

- Avoid high-fat lunchmeat, bacon, sausage, and hot dogs.
- Bake, broil, steam, or barbecue foods (no frying).
- Remove the skin of poultry and trim excess fat from meat.
- Use fat-free or low-fat (1%) milk and dairy products.
- Eat boiled beans (or low-fat refried).
- Use nonstick pans, nonstick vegetable spray, or small amounts of margarine or oil (1–2 tsp) for cooking.
- Reduce added fat in the diet, such as butter, margarine, sour cream, mayonnaise, nuts, avocados, cream, cream cheese, and salad dressings.
- Avoid high-fat and high-sugar snack foods such as chips, cookies, donuts, pie, cake, candy, and ice cream. Use low-fat snacks such as fresh vegetables, bread sticks, or pretzels.

RECORD KEEPING AND FOLLOW-UP

Ask your patient to keep accurate records of food intake, including time of meal or snack and amount eaten, blood glucose levels, and timing and dose of insulin taken. During follow-up visits, the dietitian and patient should review the food records for nutritional adequacy, appropriate weight gain, and glycemic responses to food. Evaluate the patient's understanding and compliance with the meal plan; any problem areas may then be addressed. Records are very important because they allow for the identification of individual food sensitivities. The dietitian can provide feedback on the patient's food intake and blood glucose levels. Most important, analysis of the records helps the patient make better decisions about what and how much to eat.

Dietary and/or insulin adjustments should be made in conjunction with the primary care physician, especially if problems such as hyperglycemia, hypoglycemia, and presence of urinary ketones, weight loss, or excessive weight gain are identified.

SODIUM, CAFFEINE, AND ARTIFICIAL SWEETENERS

SODIUM

The sodium requirement during pregnancy is 2,300 mg daily, the same as a non-pregnant adult woman (17).

CAFFEINE

Caffeine has not been directly linked to birth defects. Recent reports do show that large quantities of caffeine ingested (>300 mg/day) increase the risk of intrauterine growth retardation and spontaneous abortion (18). Therefore, because of potential harm to the fetus, pregnant women who consume caffeine-containing beverages should do so in moderation. The suggested limit is 300 mg caffeine daily, about the amount in two and a half cups of coffee.

ARTIFICIAL SWEETENERS

The use of artificial sweeteners in pregnancy is considered safe in moderation. Available noncaloric sweeteners include saccharin, aspartame, acesulfame-K, sucralose, and neotame (7). There are no specific recommendations concerning intake levels. Blends of artificial sweeteners that contain dextrose will affect blood glucose levels and must be counted in the meal plan.

MANAGEMENT OF HYPOGLYCEMIA

The pregnant woman who requires insulin may become hypoglycemic if she delays meals, skips a snack or meal, exercises more than usual, or takes too much insulin and eats too little food. Because all pregnant women become desensitized to low blood glucose levels, hypoglycemia unawareness is universally experienced. Thus, women cannot wait for symptoms to appear to treat low blood glucose. They must check blood glucose at those time points when hypoglycemia is most likely: 10:00 a.m., 3:00 p.m., 8:00 p.m., and 3:00 a.m. Any blood glucose level <60 mg/dl (<3.3 mmol/l) should be treated. In addition, a woman should not drive a car unless her blood glucose is >90 mg/dl (>5 mmol/l). The patient must also be counseled to self-monitor her blood glucose if she experiences symptoms of hypoglycemia, such as headache, dizziness, drowsiness, cold sweat, irritability, and difficulty speaking, in addition to her normal self-monitored blood glucose schedule.

POSTPARTUM NUTRITIONAL MANAGEMENT

The nutritional quality of a woman's diet remains very important during the postpartum period, regardless of whether she chooses to breastfeed or bottle-feed her baby. In either case, she is recovering from the physiological stresses of pregnancy and delivery as well as coping with the additional work and demands of the new baby. The patient should be encouraged to continue to follow her pregnancy meal plan or work with her dietitian to develop a new one.

Most women want to lose weight quickly after delivery and may adopt inadequate or inappropriate eating habits to do so. They may not realize the importance of replenishing nutrient stores lost during pregnancy. Weight loss should be discussed with all women shortly after delivery. Prepregnancy weight, weight gain during pregnancy, desirable weight for height, breastfeeding status, age, and exercise level should be thoroughly assessed to direct each woman to an appropriate weight loss schedule. Gradual loss of weight gained during pregnancy, as well as excess prepregnant weight, can be accomplished by exercising regularly and following a moderately hypocaloric diet aimed at a weight loss of 0.5–1 lb/week. A more rapid weight loss is not recommended because it may contribute to fatigue and nutrient depletion.

LACTATION

Breastfeeding is recommended for women with diabetes. In addition to health benefits ranging from lower breast cancer risk to an enhanced immune system, insulin requirements for diabetic nursing mothers average 25% lower during lactation, and some experience a temporary complete remission of their symptoms (19–21). Breastfeeding may be especially important to the infant of a diabetic mother, as several studies have shown a protective effect against obesity (22) and early diabetes (23,24). Although preliminary research suggests that diabetic milk may have altered composition that could predispose to obesity and impaired glucose tolerance, altogether, the benefits of mother's milk to the infant still outweigh these concerns (24–26).

ENERGY REQUIREMENTS

While breastfeeding, a woman's calorie, fluid, protein, vitamin, and mineral requirements are increased. She must meet her own postpartum nutritional needs as well as produce an adequate volume of milk to meet her baby's nutritional needs.

Among mothers exclusively breastfeeding their infants, the energy demands of lactation exceed prepregnancy demands by ~650 kcal/day, assuming milk output of 780 ml/day and including the energy used for production during the first 6 months postpartum (27,28). These needs may be partially met by extra fat stored during pregnancy, which can provide on average 150–170 kcal/day (28). Therefore, an additional 450–500 kcal/day over the prepregnant allowance may be needed, decreasing by 100 kcal during the second half-year as milk output declines (28). Individual energy needs vary depending on the volume of milk produced, the amount of stored fat, and the woman's energy expenditure (28). One study that tracked energy intake and lactation performance among type 1 diabetic mothers found that a daily prescription of 31 kcal/kg maternal body weight was associated with sustained milk production (29). The American Diabetes Association suggests that an energy intake of no less than ~1,800 kcal/day will usually meet the nursing mother's nutritional requirements for lactation while allowing for a gradual weight loss (30).

The relationship between breastfeeding and weight loss is neither consistent nor conclusive, although many women lose weight during the first 6 months of lactation. The average rate of weight loss is ~0.5–1 kg/month (~1–2 lb/month) after the first month postpartum, with 1–2 kg/month (4–5 lb) acceptable for women who are significantly overweight (31). Rapid weight loss (>2 kg/month [>4.4 lb/month] after the first month postpartum) is not advised for breastfeeding women. Intakes <1,500 kcal/day have resulted in decreased milk output (32). Liquid diets and weight loss medications are not recommended. Exercise is recommended for lactating women to reduce their body fat and increase their fitness level.

MATERNAL SUPPLEMENTATION

During the postpartum period, the need for supplementation depends on the woman's nutritional status (21,31). Women found to be anemic after delivery or at their postpartum checkup should take 60–120 mg/day of ferrous sulfate until the anemia is resolved. Nutrients most likely to be inadequate in the diet of a lactating woman in general are calcium, magnesium, zinc, thiamin, vitamin B6, and folate. Thorough dietary assessment and counseling will assist women in selecting and consuming foods that are rich in these nutrients. Although routine vitamin/mineral supplementation in lactating women is not recommended, specific nutrient supplementation may be warranted for women at nutritional risk.

CARBOHYDRATES, PROTEIN, AND GLYCEMIC CONTROL

Milk synthesis requires glucose. To meet the additional demand during lactation, the estimated average requirement (EAR) for carbohydrates is 160 g/day with an RDA of 210 g/day, while the EAR for protein is 1.05 g/kg/day with an RDA of 71 g/day (33,34).

Normoglycemic women do not appear to experience significant changes between pre- and post-breastfeeding blood glucose levels nor do they exhibit any hypoglycemic responses to lactation (35). However, blood glucose levels may be more variable during lactation for women with type 1 diabetes, and both hyper- and hypoglycemia are possible. The extent of variability may depend on the amount of milk produced and the frequency of feeding (36). Hypoglycemia may be more likely between meals; therefore, mothers may need to include snacks containing protein and carbohydrate before or during breastfeeding (37). Blood glucose should be tested more frequently to determine the need for extra snacks. To avoid hypoglycemia in the middle of the night (2:00–6:00 a.m.), the woman should eat a high-protein snack before bed, or the evening intermediate- or long-acting insulin should be decreased. Because most women experience fatigue postpartum and sleep more, there is a risk that they will sleep through a meal or snack, with resulting hypoglycemia. To avoid this, the patient should be encouraged to nap after meals and snacks, not before.

FLUID REQUIREMENTS

Contrary to popular belief, breastfeeding mothers do not need to drink large amounts of fluids to produce sufficient milk. In one study, control mothers who drank ad libitum took in ~2 liters per day while producing adequate milk for their babies' needs, whereas an experimental group forced to drink 3 liters experienced lower milk production and infant weight gain (38). Breastfeeding mothers should drink to thirst. Encouraging mothers to sip on a beverage (preferably water or caffeine-free tea) while nursing with a goal of keeping their urine a pale yellow is a good way to help them pay attention to their needs.

COURSE OF LACTATION

Diabetic mothers are at increased risk for lactation complications (21). Poor metabolic control during pregnancy can negatively affect serum prolactin as well as placental lactogen and mammary development, which can ultimately affect their milk production (39). In addition, diabetic mothers tend to have lower prolactin and higher nitrogen levels than nondiabetic mothers in the first week, which correlates with slower onset of copious milk production. Fluctuations in blood glucose levels after birth can impair lactose synthesis (40–42) and delay the onset of lactogenesis II an average of 15–28 hours (43,44). Poor glycemic control during lactation can negatively affect milk production (44), and lower infant intake has been observed, even in some euglycemic mothers (45). Concomitant thyroid dysfunctions may also interfere with lactation (46).

Hypoglycemia, respiratory distress, or other complications in the infant of a diabetic mother also can lead to supplementation and interference with the early establishment of breastfeeding. Early and frequent feedings may help to minimize neonatal hypoglycemia, but mothers at risk may desire to manually express and freeze colostrum during the last trimester to use at the hospital if supplementation becomes necessary (47). One study found an inverse relationship between delay in first suckling and duration of lactation; thus, a supportive environment that minimizes mother-infant separation may increase the probability of successful lactation (20). Although they have more difficulty in the beginning and have a higher fallout rate, those who make it past the early weeks have the same duration of breastfeeding as nondiabetic nursing mothers (48).

Diabetic mothers are also more prone to mastitis and candidal infections of the nipple/breast during lactation (44). Optimal management of diabetes minimizes such complications, and with good metabolic control, diabetic nursing mothers breastfeed as well as their nonaffected counterparts once they successfully navigate any early postpartum issues (29,48,26,49,21).

REFERENCES

1. Institute of Medicine: *Dietary References Intakes. Part 2.* Washington, DC, National Academies Press, 2002

2. Institute of Medicine: *Nutrition During Pregnancy.* Washington, DC, National Academies Press, 1990

3. Centers for Disease Control and Prevention: Spina Bifida and Anencephaly before and after folic acid mandate—United States. 1995–1996 and 1999–2000. *MMWR* 53:362–65, 2004

4. Persaud VL, Van der Hof MC, Dubé Jm, Zimmer P: Incidence of open neural tube defects in Nova Scotia after folic acid fortification. *Canadian Medical Association Journal* 167:241–45, 2002

5. Grover SR, Morley R: Vitamin D deficiency in veiled or dark-skinned women. *Med J Aust.* 175:251–52, 2001

6. Institute of Medicine: *Dietary Reference Intakes for Vitamin A, Vitamin K, Arsenic, Boron, Chromium, Copper, Iodine, Iron, Manganese, Molybdenum, Nickel, Silicon, Vanadium, and Zinc.* Food and Nutrition Board. Washington, DC, National Academy Press, 2001

7. Position of the American Dietetic Association: Nutrition and lifestyle for a healthy pregnancy outcome. *J Am Diet Assoc.* 102:1479–90, 2002

8. Stevens DL: The use of complementary alternative therapies in diabetes. *Clinics in Family Practice.* 4:191, 2002

9. Brown J, Carlson M: Nutrition and multifetal pregnancy. *J Am Diet Assoc.* 100:343–48, 2000

10. Diabetes Care and Education. *Diabetes and Pregnancy.* 28, 9, 2007

11. Peterson CM, Jovanovic-Peterson L: Percentage of carbohydrate and glycemic response to breakfast, lunch, and dinner in women with gestational diabetes. *Diabetes* 40 (Suppl. 2):172–74, 1991

12. Jovanovic-Peterson L, Peterson CM, Reed G, NICHD-DIEP: Maternal postprandial glucose levels predict birth weight. *Am F Obstet Gynecol* 164:103–11, 1991

13. American Diabetes Association: Nutrition recommendations and principles for people with diabetes mellitus. *Diabetes Care* 23 (Suppl. 1):543–46, 2000

14. Jovanovic L, Druzin M, Peterson CM: Effect of euglycemia on the outcome of pregnancy in insulin-dependent diabetic women as compared with normal control subjects. *Am F Med* 71:921–27, 1981

15. Jovanovic-Peterson L, Peterson CM: Dietary manipulation as a primary

treatment strategy for pregnancies complicated by diabetes. *F Am Coll Nutr* 9:320–25, 1990

16. California Diabetes and Pregnancy Program: *Sweet Success California Diabetes and Pregnancy Program Guidelines for Care.* Revised ed. Sacramento, CA, State of California Department of Public Health, Maternal, Child and Adolescent Health Division, 2008

17. Institute of Medicine: *Dietary Reference Intakes: The Essential Guide to Nutrient Requirements.* Washington, DC, National Academies Press, 2006

18. Cnattingius S, Signorelo LB, Anneren G, Clausson B, Ekbom A, et al.: Caffeine intake and the risk of first trimester spontaneous abortion. *N Engl J Med.* 3343:1839–45, 2000

19. Davies HA, Clark JD, Dalton KJ, Edwards OM: Insulin requirements of diabetic women who breast feed. *BMJ* 298:1357–58, 1989

20. Asselin BL, Lawrence RA: Maternal disease as a consideration in lactation management. *Clin Perinatol* 14:71–87, 1987

21. Lawrence RA, Lawrence RM: *Breastfeeding: A Guide for the Medical Profession.* 6th ed. Philadelphia, Elsevier Mosby, 2005

22. Kreichauf S, Pfluger M, Hummel S, Ziegler AG: [Effect of breastfeeding on the risk of becoming overweight in offspring of mothers with type 1 diabetes]. *Dtsch Med Wochenschr* 133:1173–77, 2008

23. Taylor JS, Kacmar JE, Nothnagle M, Lawrence RA: A systematic review of the literature associating breastfeeding with type 2 diabetes and gestational diabetes. *J Am Coll Nutr* 24:320–26, 2005

24. Kjos SL: After pregnancy complicated by diabetes: postpartum care and education. *Obstet Gynecol Clin North Am* 34:335–49, 2007

25. Plagemann A, Harder T: Breast feeding and the risk of obesity and related metabolic diseases in the child. *Metab Syndr Relat Disord* 3:222–32, 2005

26. Stage E, Norgard H, Damm P, Mathiesen E: Long-term breast-feeding in women with type 1 diabetes. *Diabetes Care* 29:771–74, 2006

27. Butte NF, King JC: Energy requirements during pregnancy and lactation. *Public Health Nutr* 8:1010–27, 2005

28. Hopkinson J: Nutrition in lactation. In *Hale and Hartmann's Textbook of Human Lactation.* 1st ed. Hale T, Hartmann P, Eds. Amarillo, TX, Hale Publishing, 2007, p. 371–86

29. Ferris AM, Dalidowitz CK, Ingardia CM, Reece EA, Fumia FD, Jensen RG, Allen LH: Lactation outcome in insulin-dependent diabetic women. *J Am Diet Assoc* 88:317–22, 1988

30. American Diabetes Association: Nutrition principles and recommendations in diabetes (Position Statement). *Diabetes Care* 27 (Suppl. 1):S36, 2004

31. Institute of Medicine: *Nutrition During Lactation.* Washington, DC, National Academies Press, 1991

32. Strode MA, Dewey KG, Lonnerdal B: Effects of short-term caloric restriction on lactational performance of well-nourished women. *Acta Paediatr Scand* 75:222–29, 1986

33. Food and Nutrition Board: *Dietary Reference Intakes.* Washington, DC, National Academies Press, 2004

34. Reader D, Franz MJ: Lactation, diabetes, and nutrition recommendations. *Curr Diab Rep* 4:370–76, 2004

35. Bentley-Lewis R, Goldfine AB, Green DE, Seely EW: Lactation after normal pregnancy is not associated with blood glucose fluctuations. *Diabetes Care* 30:2792–93, 2007

36. Murtaugh MA, Ferris AM, Capacchione CM, Reece EA: Energy intake and glycemia in lactating women with type 1 diabetes. *J Am Diet Assoc* 98:642–48, 1998

37. Bradley C: Managing diabetes while breast-feeding. *Diabetes Self Manag* 24:84, 87–89, 2007

38. Illingworth RS, Kilpatrick B: Lactation and fluid intake. *Lancet* 2:1175–77, 1953

39. Neubauer SH: Lactation in insulin-dependent diabetes. *Prog Food Nutr Sci* 14:333–70, 1990

40. Arthur PG, Kent JC, Hartmann PE: Metabolites of lactose synthesis in milk from diabetic and nondiabetic women during lactogenesis II. *J Pediatr Gastroenterol Nutr* 19:100–08, 1994

41. Oliveira AM, da Cunha CC, Penha-Silva N, Abdallah VO, Jorge PT: [Interference of the blood glucose control in the transition between phases I and II of lactogenesis in patients with type 1 diabetes mellitus]. *Arq Bras Endocrinol Metabol* 52:473–81, 2008

42. Hartmann P, Cregan M: Lactogenesis and the effects of insulin-dependent diabetes mellitus and prematurity. *J Nutr* 131:3016S–20S, 2001

43. Arthur PG, Smith M, Hartmann PE: Milk lactose, citrate, and glucose as markers of lactogenesis in normal and diabetic women. *J Pediatr Gastroenterol Nutr* 9:488–96, 1989

44. Neubauer SH, Ferris AM, Chase CG, Fanelli J, Thompson CA, Lammi-Keefe CJ, Clark RM, Jensen RG, Bendel RB, Green KW: Delayed lactogenesis in women with insulin-dependent diabetes mellitus. *Am J Clin Nutr* 58:54–60, 1993

45. Miyake A, Tahara M, Koike K, Tanizawa O: Decrease in neonatal suckled milk volume in diabetic women. *Eur J Obstet Gynecol Reprod Biol* 33:49–53, 1989

46. Marasco L: The impact of thyroid dysfunction on lactation. *Breastfeeding Abstracts* 25:9, 11–12, 2006

47. Cox S: Expressing and storing colostrum antenatally for use in the newborn period. *Breastfeeding Review* 14:5–8, 2006

48. Ferris AM, Neubauer SH, Bendel RB, Green KW, Ingardia CJ, Reece EA: Perinatal lactation protocol and outcome in mothers with and without insulin-dependent diabetes mellitus. *Am J Clin Nutr* 58:43–48, 1993

49. Walker M: Maternal acute and chronic illness. In *Core Curriculum for Lactation Consultant Practice*. 2nd ed. Mannel R, Martens P, Walker M, Eds. Sudbury, MA, Jones and Bartlett, 2007, p. 690–91

SUGGESTED READING

American Dietetic Association: *Nutrition Practice Guidelines for Gestational Diabetes Mellitus: ADA MNT Evidence-Based Guides for Practice*. Chicago, American Dietetic Association, 2001

Centers for Disease Control and Prevention: Spina bifida and anencephaly before and after folic acid mandate: United States, 1995–1996 and 1999–2000. *MMWR* 53:362–65, 2004

Dewey KG, McCrory MA: Effects of dieting and physical activity on pregnancy and lactation. *Am J Clin Nutr* 59:446S–52S, 1994

Feig DS, Briggs GG, Koren G: Oral antidiabetic agents in pregnancy and lactation: a paradigm shift? *Ann Pharmacother* 41:1174–80, 2007

Gunderson EP: Breastfeeding after gestational diabetes pregnancy: subsequent obesity and type 2 diabetes in women and their offspring. *Diabetes Care* 30 (Suppl. 2):S161–68, 2007

Kaiser L, Allen LH, American Dietetic Association: Position of the American Dietetic Association: nutrition and lifestyle for a healthy pregnancy outcome. *J Am Diet Assoc* 108:553–61, 2008

Kjos SL: Postpartum care of the woman with diabetes. *Clin Obstet Gynecol* 43:75–86, 2000

Mayer-Davis EJ, Rifas-Shiman SL, Zhou L, Hu FB, Colditz GA, Gillman MW: Breast-feeding and risk for childhood obesity: does maternal diabetes or obesity status matter? *Diabetes Care* 29:2231–37, 2006

Murphy S, Wilson C: Breastfeeding promotion: a rational and achievable target for a type 2 diabetes prevention intervention in Native American communities. *J Hum Lact* 24:193–98, 2008

Picciano MF: Pregnancy and lactation: physiological adjustments, nutritional requirements and the role of dietary supplements. *J Nutr* 133:1997S–2002S, 2003

Rodekamp E, Harder T, Kohlhoff R, Franke K, Dudenhausen JW, Plagemann A: Long-term impact of breast-feeding on body weight and glucose tolerance in children of diabetic mothers: role of the late neonatal period and early infancy. *Diabetes Care* 28:1457–62, 2005

Rogers LM, Jovanovic L, Becker DJ: Should she or shouldn't she? The relationship between infant feeding practices and type 1 diabetes in the genetically at risk. *Diabetes Care* 28:2809, 2005

Schaefer-Graf UM, Hartmann R, Pawliczak J, Passow D, Abou-Dakn M, Vetter K, Kordonouri O: Association of breast-feeding and early childhood overweight in children from mothers with gestational diabetes mellitus. *Diabetes Care* 29:1105–07, 2006

Talim M: Breast-feeding and risk for childhood obesity: response to Mayer-Davis et al. *Diabetes Care* 30:451, 2007

Walker M: Breastfeeding with diabetes: yes you can! *J Hum Lact* 22:345–46, 2006

Webster J, Moore K, Dip G, McMullan A, Nurs B: Breastfeeding outcomes for women with insulin dependent diabetes. *J Hum Lact* 11:195–200, 1995

Whichelow MJ, Doddridge MC: Lactation in diabetic women. *Br Med J (Clin Res Ed)* 287:649, 1983

Ziegler A-G, Schmid S, Huber D, Hummel M, Bonifacio E: Early infant feeding and risk of developing type 1 diabetes-associated autoantibodies. *JAMA* 290:1721–28, 2003

Use of Insulin During Pregnancy in Preexisting Diabetes

Highlights
Use of Insulin During Pregnancy in Preexisting Diabetes

■ The metabolic alterations in early pregnancy include loss of glucose and gluconeogenic substrates, which can lead to hypoglycemia, especially during the night.

■ During midgestation, insulin requirements begin to increase as the woman changes to a lipid-based energy economy.

■ In late gestation, insulin resistance due to placental production of contrainsulin hormones results in even greater insulin requirements.

■ Postpartum insulin injections may not be necessary for as long as 48–72 h because of release of insulin stores created prepartum. Insulin need must be recalculated using postpartum weight and plans for diet, exercise, and breastfeeding.

■ To deal with these metabolic changes and maintain normal blood glucose levels, the pregnant diabetic woman must perform frequent self-monitoring of blood glucose, and she and her health care team must be equipped to make immediate dosage adjustments in response to each measurement.

■ A multiple-injection routine is necessary to replicate normal meal-stimulated insulin output during pregnancy. The use of insulin pumps may be appropriate.

■ To prepare for active labor, when insulin requirements disappear and glucose requirements remain relatively constant, target glucose levels of 70–90 mg/dl (3.9–5.0 mmol/l) should be maintained.

Use of Insulin During Pregnancy in Preexisting Diabetes

METABOLIC ALTERATIONS DURING NORMAL GESTATION

During pregnancy, metabolism adapts to meet maternal needs and to provide fuel for the growing fetoplacental unit (1). Beginning in early gestation, glucose reaches the fetus by facilitated diffusion—it crosses the placenta at a rate faster than would be predicted physiologically. Similarly, amino acids are actively transported to the fetal circulation against a concentration gradient. Of particular importance is a decrease in the maternal plasma concentration of the gluconeogenic amino acid alanine.

Loss of glucose and gluconeogenic substrate to the fetus occurs concomitantly and conspires to cause maternal hypoglycemia during early pregnancy. Toward the end of the first trimester, it is common for insulin requirements in women with type 1 diabetes to diminish by 10–20% of the dosage taken before conception. Moreover, blood glucose control during the first trimester is more unstable than usual, and nocturnal hypoglycemia is especially common.

At 18–24 wk of gestation, the so-called diabetogenic stress of pregnancy begins, and daily insulin requirement typically begins to increase. At this time, the mother switches from a primarily glucose-based to a lipid-based energy economy derived from either circulating fats or stored adipose tissue to spare glucose for fetal growth.

In late pregnancy, basal insulin levels are higher than normal nongravid levels, and eating produces a two- to threefold greater outpouring of insulin (insulin requirement is usually 0.9–1.2 U/kg/24 h [0.4–0.6 U/lb/24 h]). These increases in plasma insulin are opposed by diminished responsiveness to insulin action due to placental production of contrainsulin hormones—human placental lactogen, prolactin, estrogen, and progesterone—and increased maternal production of cortisol.

During the second and third trimesters, insulin requirements gradually increase to as much as twice the total daily dosage of insulin needed before pregnancy. Placental growth and the production of contrainsulin hormones plateau at ~36 wk. As a result, the dosage of insulin necessary to maintain euglycemia increases very little, if at all, from 36 wk until term. A decrease in insulin requirement after 36 wk should not necessarily be interpreted as an indication of a failing fetoplacental unit.

After delivery of the placenta, human placental lactogen, estrogen, and progesterone rapidly clear from the circulation. Pituitary growth hormone and gonadotropin remain suppressed, despite the falling placental hormones. The result is a state of "panhypopituitarism." In addition, high prepartum doses of insulin create stores of bound insulin that continue to be released, whereas the need for insulin diminishes. Therefore, it is sometimes unnecessary to resume subcutaneous insulin injections for as long as 48–72 h postpartum. The dosage of insulin required postpartum must be recalculated based on postpartum weight, diet, exercise, and plans for breastfeeding.

Understanding the marked metabolic alterations in normal pregnancies and pregnancies complicated by diabetes leads to several important clinical generalizations:

- Hyperglycemia exerts potentially devastating effects on the fetus throughout pregnancy and therefore must be avoided.
- Nongravid criteria cannot be used to assess metabolism during pregnancy. Therefore, separate standards must be used to monitor diabetes management (2).
- Women with type 1 diabetes require frequent (eight times per day; see page 51) self-monitoring of blood glucose (SMBG) throughout gestation to promptly recognize the need for adjustments of their insulin dosage.
- Multiple injections of insulin are necessary to truly replicate the qualitative and quantitative changes in normal meal-related insulin output.

THERAPEUTIC INSULIN USE

The primary goal of insulin replacement is to achieve plasma glucose concentrations nearly identical to those observed in nondiabetic women. However, the goal of rigid glycemic control should not be maintained at the cost of symptomatic hypoglycemia. Therapy must be individualized and the changing insulin requirements at various stages of gestation anticipated.

INSULIN REGIMENS

Human insulins are the least immunogenic of all insulins and should be used exclusively during pregnancy. Various insulin preparations may be used in combination to achieve optimal glycemic control. The proper use of insulin requires an understanding of the factors that affect its absorption, disposal, and action. Table 21 lists the onset, peak, and duration of action of the most commonly used types of insulin.

A single daily injection of intermediate-acting (NPH) and short-acting (regular) insulin does not provide adequate insulin replacement to ensure satisfactory 24-h glycemic control. Most women with type 1 diabetes require three or more daily injections (3,4). Now that we have available safe, rapid-achieving insulins, the optimal multiple injection schedule is three injections of NPH and three injections of a rapid-acting analog.

A two-injection regimen can cause nocturnal hypoglycemic episodes if the intermediate-acting insulin given before the evening meal exerts its peak action during the middle of the night. Thus, the mixtures of 70/30 or 75/25 given before dinner should be avoided. Patients should set an alarm clock and perform SMBG at 0300 or 0400. Fitful sleep, profuse sweating, nightmares, or morning headaches suggest nocturnal hypoglycemia. Note that fasting hyperglycemia may signify a middle-of-the-night low. To eliminate the problem of nocturnal hypoglycemia, the

Table 23 Insulins by Comparative Action

	Onset (h)	Peak (h)	Effective duration (h)
Rapid acting [manufacturer]			
Insulin lispro (analog) [Lilly]	<0.3–0.5	0.5–2.5	3–6.5
Insulin aspart (analog) [Novo Nordisk]	<0.25	0.5–1	3–5
Insulin glulisine (analog) [Sanofi Aventis]	<0.25	1–1.5	3–5
Short acting			
Regular (soluble) [Lilly, Novo Nordisk]	0.5–1	2–3	3–6
Intermediate acting			
NPH (isophane) [Lilly, Novo Nordisk]	2–4	4–10	10–16
Long acting			
Insulin glargine (analog) [Aventis]	2–4	Relatively flat	20–24
Insulin detemir (analog) [Novo Nordisk]	0.8–2 (dose dependent)	Relatively flat	Dose dependent; 12 h for 0.2 U/kg; 20 h for 0.4 U/kg, up to 24 h. Binds to albumin.
Combinations			
50% NPH, 50% regular [Lilly]	0.5–1	Dual	10–16
70% NPH, 30% regular [Lilly]	0.5–1	Dual	10–16
75% NPL, 25% lispro [Lilly]	<0.25	Dual	10–16
50% NPL, 50% lispro [Lilly]	<0.25	Dual	10–16
70% aspart protamine, 30% aspart [Novo Nordisk]	<0.25	Dual	15–18

evening dose of intermediate-acting insulin should be delayed until bedtime so that its peak action coincides with breakfast the next morning. In any regimen that includes a morning dose of rapid- and intermediate-acting insulins, lunch must be constant in composition and timing.

Greater precision of insulin administration and more flexibility can be achieved with multiple injections of rapid-acting insulin before each meal and intermediate-acting insulin given every 8 h to mimic the physiological secretion of basal insulin. Regimens that include multiple preprandial injections of rapid-acting insulin provide a degree of meal flexibility that is advantageous for pregnant women. These programs permit frequent adjustment of rapid-acting insulin to prevent hypoglycemia, particularly during the first trimester, when nausea and anorexia may be common. Patients must frequently perform SMBG and learn to anticipate insulin needs based on the content of the upcoming meal, the preprandial blood glucose, and the anticipated level of exercise. Generally, blood glucose should be measured eight times daily (before and after each meal, at bedtime, and in the middle of the night).

There are sufficient data accruing on the rapid-acting insulin analogs insulin lispro and insulin aspart, and these data were used by the experts at the Fifth International Workshop-Conference on Gestational Diabetes Mellitus to advocate the use of these drugs in pregnancy. To date, there are no clinical trials showing the safety and efficacy of insulin glargine, insulin detemir, or insulin glulisine in pregnancy (5).

INSULIN PUMPS

On the premise that the ultimate glycemic control is to mimic normal pancreatic insulin release, some clinicians have recommended continuous subcutaneous insulin infusion via an insulin pump (6). Insulin pumps deliver a basal rate of insulin infusion with pulse-dose increments before meals. They have been used safely and successfully during pregnancy.

Most people will require at least three infusion rates: 2400–0400, 0400–1000, and 1000–2400. The lowest basal dose is usually administered at 2400–0400. From 0400 to 1000, cortisol and growth hormone levels rise, and the basal rate of insulin must be increased. The progressive increase in contrainsulin hormones accompanying pregnancy will require a corresponding increase in basal infusion rate. If the basal infusion rate is properly calculated, glucose concentrations will be perfect during fasting, and each meal or snack will require a bolus of insulin. A detailed protocol for calculating basal infusion rates and bolus doses has been described by Jovanovic-Peterson and Peterson (7).

DOSAGE ADJUSTMENT

Patients must be encouraged to check blood glucose levels frequently and record the results in a form that permits recognition of glycemic patterns. Patients and their health care team often immediately adjust the dosage of insulin in response to every serum glucose measurement that lies outside the target range. This reactive approach to blood glucose control should be avoided. The essential principles for any successful insulin regimen include observation of glucose patterns and gradual prospective dosage adjustments.

For example, a patient experiencing elevated blood glucose concentrations during the late afternoon should not react by giving supplemental insulin before dinner and risking hypoglycemia later in the evening. Instead, she should plan to increase her morning dose of intermediate-acting insulin the next morning (if she is taking a mixed morning dose) or to increase her noon dose of rapid-acting insulin. In another case, a woman with satisfactory fasting blood glucose but low midmorning and midafternoon values can often eliminate both episodes of hypoglycemia by reducing the morning dose of short-acting insulin without altering the dose of intermediate-acting insulin. The effect of the rapid-acting insulin that lowered the midmorning glucose disappeared by afternoon but set the stage for the peak action of intermediate-acting insulin to cause an insulin reaction.

However, there are exceptions. For example, a hypoglycemic reaction that cannot be explained by a missed meal or increased exercise should be followed by a reduction in the next dose. Similarly, algorithms for controlling blood glucose on sick days may require the addition of 1 or 2 U short-acting insulin in response to preprandial hyperglycemia.

INSULIN USE FOR PRETERM DELIVERY

Preterm delivery can be particularly hazardous and presents a special therapeutic dilemma in diabetic pregnancy (see also page 141). β-Sympathomimetics, the most commonly used tocolytic agents, are capable of causing rapid and extreme elevations in maternal glucose concentration and possibly ketoacidosis. Corticosteroids, used to accelerate fetal lung maturation, can further exacerbate hyperglycemia. However, if no attempt is made to halt preterm labor, respiratory distress syndrome in the premature infant may result. The following protocol may be used to adjust insulin dosage when corticosteroids are needed to enhance fetal lung maturity:

- Give 12 mg dexamethasone orally on two successive mornings.
- During the 2 days of steroid therapy, double the total daily dosage of insulin.
- Check blood glucose concentration every 4 h, and give supplemental short-acting insulin as needed.

Tocolytic therapy should only be undertaken in centers where continuous, experienced maternal-fetal supervision is available. Throughout parenteral tocolytic therapy, maternal glucose should initially be measured hourly and every 2–4 h once blood glucose is stable. Use of continuous infusion of the β-mimetic minimizes the hyperglycemic response. In some patients, tocolysis can be achieved with medications less likely to cause hyperglycemia (e.g., magnesium sulfate or indomethacin).

INSULIN DURING LABOR AND DELIVERY

Intrapartum glycemic control plays a major role in the well-being of the neonate. Maternal hyperglycemia is the major cause of neonatal hypoglycemia. At the onset of active labor, insulin requirements decrease to zero, and glucose requirements are relatively constant at ~2.5 mg/kg/min (1.1 mg/lb/min) (8,9). From these data, Jovanovic and Peterson (7–9) developed a protocol for meeting the glucose needs of active labor. The goal is to maintain a plasma glucose concentration between 70 and 90 mg/dl (3.9 and 5.0 mmol/l).

- On the evening before elective induction, the usual bedtime dose of intermediate-acting insulin may be given.
- On the morning of induction, insulin is withheld and an intravenous infusion of normal saline begun.
- Once active labor commences or plasma glucose level falls to <70 mg/dl (<3.9 mmol/l), normal saline should be changed to 5% dextrose and infused at a rate of 2.5 mg/kg/min or ~10 g/kg/h (1.1 mg/lb/min or ~4.6 g/lb/h).
- Glucose level should be monitored hourly, and if it is <60 mg/dl (<3.3 mmol/l), the infusion rate should be doubled for the subsequent hour.
- If the plasma glucose concentration rises to >140 mg/dl (>7.8 mmol/l), 2–4 U intravenous human regular or subcutaneous rapid-acting insulin can be given each hour until the glucose value is in the range of 70–90 mg/dl (3.9–5.0 mmol/l).

With elective cesarean delivery,

■ The bedtime dose of intermediate-acting insulin may be given on the morning of surgery and every 8 h if surgery is delayed.
■ A dextrose infusion as described above may be started if the glucose concentration falls to <60 mg/dl (<3.3 mmol/l).
■ Alternatively, glycemic control before elective cesarean delivery can be achieved with an infusion of 1–2 U/h intravenous human regular or subcutaneous rapid-acting insulin given simultaneously with 5 g/h dextrose. The insulin infusion should be discontinued immediately before surgery.
■ Hourly blood glucose determinations are mandatory to allow for individualization of these protocols.

See Table 22.

POSTPARTUM INSULIN REQUIREMENTS

After delivery, insulin requirements diminish precipitously. As a result, it is often unnecessary to administer subcutaneous insulin for 24–72 h. Insulin requirements should be recalculated at 0.6 U/kg/24 h (2.7 U/lb/24 h), based on postpartum weight and should be started when either postprandial or fasting glucose is >150 mg/dl (>8.3 mmol/l).

BREASTFEEDING

There are few data on the changes in insulin requirements necessary to maintain good metabolic control while breastfeeding. Several investigators have reported that patterns of glucose control may be erratic in lactating diabetic women. Episodes of hypoglycemia appear to be common. Recommendations for lactating mothers include increasing calorie intake while maintaining the decreased postpartum insulin dosage (see page 83).

The optimal insulin program varies for each patient, and SMBG should provide the data necessary to adjust the dosage and timing of insulin injections. Because hypoglycemia is most likely to occur within an hour after breastfeeding, this is an important time to measure blood glucose. In most cases, hypoglycemia can be avoided by eating a small snack before breastfeeding rather than making frequent adjustments of the insulin dosage (10). Nocturnal hypoglycemia is particularly common. Therefore, blood glucose should be periodically checked during the night, and the evening dose of intermediate-acting insulin should be decreased if hypoglycemia is documented (10–12).

ORAL HYPOGLYCEMIC AGENTS

In the United States, oral hypoglycemic agents are contraindicated for use during pregnancy. Although there are no published controlled studies, isolated reports of human teratogenesis exist. These agents have recently been reported to be safe for gestational diabetes, but no study to date proves that they are safe or efficacious in the treatment of pre–gestational diabetes.

Table 22 Two Protocols for Insulin Management of Labor and Delivery

The usual dose of intermediate-acting insulin is given at bedtime, but the usual morning dose is withheld. In both protocols the glucose levels are checked hourly using a bedside meter allowing for adjustment in the insulin or glucose infusion rate. The protocols differ in the BG thresholds at which to infuse dextrose-containing solutions and at which to infuse Regular short-acting insulin. Many nursing clinicians believe it is simpler to always infuse 5% dextrose, as with perioperative management of diabetic patients. Data discussed in the text suggest a maternal glucose target <100 mg/dL (<5.6 mmol/l) to minimize neonatal hypoglycemia. Protocol A is taken ACOG05a based on data from (12) and (6); protocol B is taken from (13) and assumes that many patients with DM1 will have a small insulin requirement to remain normoglycemic. LR, lactated Ringer's solution; D5LR, 5% dextrose lactated Ringer's solution.

	A.	**B.**
Intravenous fluids	• Intravenous infusion of normal saline is begun.	• BG >130mg/dL, LR at 125 ml/hr
	• Once active labor begins or glucose levels decrease to <70mg/dL, the infusion is changed to 5% dextrose and delivered at a rate of 100–150 cc/hr to to achieve a glucose level of ~100 mg/dL (5.6 mmol/l).	• BG <130mg/dL, begin D5LR at 125 ml/hr
Initiating insulin	• Regular (short-acting) insulin is administered by intravenous infusion at a rate of 1.25 U/hr if glucose levels exceed 100 mg/dL	• Mix 25 U Regular insulin in 250 mL normal saline (1 U: 10 mL)
		• Algorithm (see below)

Protocol B Algorithm

Maternal plasma glucose in mg/dL (mmol/l)	Insulin (U/hr)	Individualized dose
<70 (<3.9)	0	
71–90 (3.9–5.0)	0.5	
91-110 (5.1–6.1)	1	
111-130 (6.2–7.2)	2	
131-150 (7.3–8.3)	3	
151-170 (8.4–9.4)	4	
171–190 (9.5–10.6)	5	
>190 (>10.6)	Check ketones	

Sulfonylureas, cross the placenta and would be expected to increase fetal insulin production. Because hyperinsulinism contributes to abnormal fetal growth, use of these drugs is at least theoretically inappropriate. Moreover, severe prolonged hypoglycemia has been reported in the neonates of women treated with oral agents near the time of delivery (14).

REFERENCES

1. Freinkel N: Banting Lecture 1980: of pregnancy and progeny. *Diabetes* 29:1023–35, 1980

2. Freinkel N, Phelps R, Metzger BE: The mother in pregnancies complicated by diabetes. In *Diabetes Mellitus. Theory and Practice.* 4th ed. Rifkin H, Porte D Jr, Eds. New York, Elsevier, 1990, p. 634–50

3. Hare JW: *Diabetes Complicating Pregnancy: The Joslin Clinic Method.* New York, Liss, 1989

4. Jovanovic L, Peterson CM: Optimal insulin delivery for the pregnant diabetic patient. *Diabetes Care* 5 (Suppl. 1):24–35, 1982

5. Jovanovic L, Pettitt DJ: Treatment with insulin and its analogs in pregnancy complicated by diabetes. *Diabetes Care* 30:S220–24, 2007

6. Coustan DR, Reece EA, Sherwin RS, Rudolf MCJ, Bates SE, Sockin SM, Holford T, Tamborlane WV: A randomized clinical trial of the insulin pump vs. intensive conventional therapy in diabetic pregnancies. *JAMA* 255:631–36, 1986

7. Jovanovic-Peterson L, Peterson CM: Planting the pump. *Diabetes Prof* Spring:23–27, 1990

8. Jovanovic L, Peterson CM: Insulin and glucose requirements during the first stage of labor in insulin-dependent diabetic women. *Am J Med* 75:607–12, 1983

9. Jovanovic L: Glucose and insulin requirements during labor and delivery: the case for normoglycemia in pregnancies complicated by diabetes. *Endocr Pract* 10:40–45, 2004

10. Ferris AM, Reece EA: Postpartum management and lactation. In *Diabetes Mellitus in Pregnancy: Principles and Practice.* New York, Churchill Livingstone, 1988, p. 623–33

11. Jovanovic-Peterson L, Peterson CM: Maternal milk and plasma glucose and insulin levels: studies in normal and diabetic subjects. *J Am Coll Nutr* 8:125–31, 1989

12. Jovanovic L, Peterson CM, Saxena BB, Dawood MY, Saudek CD: Feasibility of maintaining normal glucose profiles in insulin-dependent pregnant diabetic women. *Am J Med* 1980 Jan;68(1):105–12

13. Kitzmiller JL, Gavin LA, Gin GD, Jovanovic-Peterson L, Main EK, Zigrang WD: Preconception care of diabetes. Glycemic control prevents congenital anomalies. *J Am Med Assoc* 265(6):731–36, 1991

14. Kemball ML, McIver C, Milner RD, Nourse CH, Schiff D, Tiernan JR: Neonatal hypoglycaemia in infants of diabetic mothers given sulphonylurea drugs in pregnancy. *Arch Dis Child* 45:696–70, 1970

Diagnostic Testing and Fetal Surveillance

Highlights
Diagnostic Testing and
Fetal Surveillance

■ Ultrasound is useful in determining gestational age, evaluating fetal anatomy, assessing fetal growth and weight, and determining fetal performance during an antepartum biophysical profile.

■ Maternal serum α-fetoprotein testing can determine open fetal defects near 16 wk of gestation.

■ Genetic tests such as amniocentesis and chorionic villus sampling can be used to detect many inherited disorders, so genetic counseling must first determine which disorders the tests should examine. Amniocentesis can also be used to determine lung maturity, which can assist in identifying fetuses at risk for respiratory distress syndrome if delivered preterm.

■ Antepartum fetal status can be determined through evaluation of the fetal heart rate. Antepartum tests have reduced the necessity for preterm delivery of infants of diabetic mothers.

■ The use of tocolytic agents to suppress preterm labor in diabetic women and corticosteroids to accelerate lung maturation of the fetus should be approached with extreme caution. Careful consideration of maternal metabolism should include emphasis on frequent blood glucose sampling and insulin infusion.

Diagnostic Testing and Fetal Surveillance

D iagnostic testing and fetal surveillance include various forms of testing performed during pregnancy to assess the normalcy and development of the fetus (Table 23). Each mode of testing is described in the order in which it is usually applied as pregnancy progresses. It is important that both caregivers and patients understand that no test exists that can ensure the birth of a perfectly normal baby. One can only look for known problems with specific tests. Therefore, no assurance can be made that "everything will be fine," no matter how many normal test results are reported.

DIAGNOSTIC TESTING WITH ULTRASOUND

Ultrasonography has widespread application in obstetrics, particularly in evaluation and management of the high-risk pregnancy. Because accurate dating of pregnancy is critical in planning various evaluations and interventions, the earliest application of ultrasound is its use in establishing correct gestational age.

Before ~7.5 wk of menstrual age (time elapsed since the first day of the last menstrual period), using standard transabdominal ultrasound equipment, the presence or absence of a gestational sac and fetal pole can be demonstrated. Between 7 and 10–12 wk of gestation, the crown-rump length of the fetus can be measured, yielding 95% confidence limits of ±4.7 days for one measurement. If multiple measurements are taken, the accuracy is increased.

Between 12 and 24 wk of gestation, dating is usually accomplished by measurement of the biparietal diameter of the fetal head and/or the fetal femur length. For these measurements, the accuracy is considerably higher at 12–20 wk (95% confidence interval ±8 days) than at 20–24 wk (95% confidence interval ±2 wk). For this reason, if ultrasound-estimated gestational age is within such confidence intervals based on last menstrual period, it is customary not to change the estimated date of delivery, assuming that the patient is relatively certain about her last menstrual period and that her menses follow a fairly consistent pattern. After 28 wk of gestation, ultrasound estimates of gestational age diminish in reliability because of the large week-to-week overlap in the measurements taken (1–6).

Once gestational age has been established, ultrasound can also be quite useful in evaluating fetal anatomy. As described elsewhere in this book, the presence of maternal diabetes carries with it a significant increase in the likelihood of major congenital malformations. Although not all such malformations can be diagnosed with ultrasound, many can be found with a thorough fetal evaluation. The likeli-

Table 23 Diagnostic Testing and Fetal Surveillance

Test	Purpose	Optimal Gestational Age (wk)	Comments
Ultrasound	Establish correct gestational age	After 7.5	7–12 wk, very accurate; 15–28 wk, accuracy ±2 wk; >28 wk, not reliable
	Screen for structural anomalies		Only detects major anomalies (spinal, cardiac) but cannot guarantee normalcy
	Determine macrosomia and polyhydramnios	28 to term	Indications of fetal effects of maternal diabetes
α-Fetoprotein	Detect open fetal defect	16	High: possible open fetal anomaly Low: possible chromosomal aneuploidy
Genetic testing	Test for Tay-Sachs, sickle cell disease, thalassemia		Can be performed in both parents before marriage in couples at risk
Genetic amniocentesis	Test for chromosomal abnormalities	16	Small risk of complications; diabetes does not increase risk of chromosomal abnormalities
Chorionic villus sampling	Test for chromosomal abnormalities	8–10	Increased rate of miscarriage
Fetal activity	Screen for fetal well-being	32–40	Simple, inexpensive
Nonstress	Screen for fetal well-being	35–40*	False-positive results in a sleeping, immature, or normal fetus
Biophysical	Evaluate chronic and acute fetal problems via ultrasound	35–40*	May be the most reliable profile
Amniocentesis	Optimize delivery timing for lung maturity	32–37	Before nonemergency induction of labor or cesarean section

*Depending on clinical situation

hood of finding abnormalities that are present increases if the a priori risk is known to be high, because the ultrasonographer is highly motivated in such cases to continue scanning until he or she is satisfied that no lesions can be found. Therefore, anatomic ultrasound studies (also known as level II ultrasound or directed ultrasound) should be carried out in diabetic pregnancies where other risk factors are known to be present. Such risk factors include an elevated glycohemoglobin level at the time of first prenatal visit, high or low serum or amniotic fluid α-fetoprotein (AFP) (see below), or suggestive past history or family history of delivering a malformed infant. Although such scans can be performed in pregnancies without any of these risk factors, the sensitivity is likely to be reduced, and a negative result in no way guarantees fetal normalcy. Patients should be informed of these limitations before scanning.

AFP TESTING

AFP, a fetal product that appears in both amniotic fluid and maternal circulation, is often present in increased concentration when an open fetal defect occurs (i.e., spinal defect or ventral wall defect, such as omphalocele or gastroschisis). Its maternal concentration may be low in some cases of chromosomal aneuploidy (i.e., trisomy 21). AFP screening is best done at ~16 wk of gestation because that is the time when it is most accurate.

Because maternal type 1 diabetes is associated with an increased risk for the defects named above, among others, maternal serum AFP (MSAFP) screening is generally offered to such patients. The MSAFP level is expressed by the laboratory in multiples of the median (MOMs) to standardize the results. Various centers recommend further testing at levels ≥2.0 or >2.5 MOMs. Women with type 1 diabetes have been reported to manifest lower MSAFP levels at a given gestational age compared with nondiabetic women. Some studies have linked this lowering of MSAFP to poor metabolic control as manifested by elevated glycohemoglobin levels. Depending on the circumstances and patient preference, an elevated MSAFP may prompt either an amniocentesis (to measure amniotic fluid AFP) or a level II ultrasound examination.

Recently, some centers have begun to offer "multiple-marker screening," in which measurements of the levels of substances other than AFP, such as human chorionic gonadatropin (hCG) and estriol, are made to improve the predictive value from chromosomal aneuploidies. Because maternal diabetes does not appear to increase the risk for such aneuploidies in the fetus, these multiple-marker tests should be considered equally appropriate for diabetic patients as for the general population.

GENETIC TESTING

Maternal diabetes does not increase the risk for genetically inherited diseases. However, individuals with diabetes, like all prenatal patients, should be questioned about family history, including ethnic background, with an eye toward the identification of a high genetic risk. For example, patients of Ashkenazi Jewish or French Canadian descent are at increased risk of being carriers for Tay-Sachs disease, a uniformly fatal autosomal recessive disorder. In addition, maternal age is associated with an increased risk for chromosomal abnormalities. Mothers over the age of 35 yr (diabetes does not change the age at which the risk increases) have an ~1/200 chance of delivering a baby with a chromosomal abnormality; about half of these babies have Down's syndrome. The general population risk is ~1/1,000. Thus, any patients for whom age or family history suggest increased genetic risk should receive thorough genetic counseling.

Genetic amniocentesis, the most common method of genetic testing, is a procedure in which a needle is inserted transabdominally into the amniotic sac with ultrasound guidance to obtain amniotic fluid. Fetal cells separated from the amniotic fluid are grown in tissue culture for karyotyping (chromosome analysis) or other types of testing. This test is generally performed at ≥14 wk of gestation, and the results may take from 2 to 4 wk to return, depending on the tests desired and the laboratory facilities. Several different enzymatic defects can also be determined on fetal cells from amniotic fluid, but each requires the services of a specialized laboratory. Thus, it is necessary to know whether a particular couple is at risk for a particular genetic disease; there is no "screening" test on amniotic fluid that can detect all of the possible genetic diseases. When amniotic fluid is withdrawn for genetic testing, AFP is usually measured as well. There is a small but definite risk of an untoward event such as premature labor, rupture of the membranes, or fetal injury associated with amniocentesis, and patients should be informed of this before the procedure.

Chorionic villus sampling (CVS), another method of obtaining tissue for genetic studies, involves taking a "biopsy" of the placenta, either via a catheter inserted into the uterus transvaginally or with a needle inserted transabdominally. A relatively new procedure, CVS is available only in specialized centers. Its advantages include the facts that it can be accomplished earlier in pregnancy than amniocentesis, at 8–10 wk, and that the results can be available in just a few days. For some couples, this decreases decision-making pressure, because first-trimester pregnancy terminations are safer and less traumatic to the mother. The primary disadvantage of CVS is that there is an increased pregnancy loss rate reported compared with amniocentesis, and a few case series have reported an excess of limb defects in the offspring, particularly with very early CVS and with inexperienced operators. Thus, couples interested in CVS should be referred to experienced centers and should undergo extensive counseling before the procedure.

FETAL SURVEILLANCE WITH ULTRASOUND

In addition to verifying gestational age and detecting major anatomic abnormalities in the fetus, ultrasound is a useful tool for the assessment of fetal growth and the estimation of fetal weight. Because the fetus of a diabetic mother may be macrosomic (large for gestational age) or alternatively may be growth retarded (small for gestational age), particularly in the presence of maternal vascular disease or hypertension, it is useful to perform periodic measurements of fetal growth during the third trimester. Excessive amounts of amniotic fluid (polyhydramnios) may also complicate diabetic pregnancy and can usually be detected with ultrasound (1–6).

FETAL ACTIVITY DETERMINATIONS

Because a diminution of the frequency or intensity of fetal movement may be associated with fetal jeopardy, many centers instruct pregnant women (particularly those with high-risk pregnancies) to "track" fetal movement daily during the third trimester. Numerous systems are used, including the recording of the number of perceived fetal movements during a given period or the recording of the amount of time that elapses until a given number of movements are perceived. Whenever preset thresholds for fetal movement are not met, the patient is asked to come in for more sophisticated biophysical antepartum testing (see below).

ANTEPARTUM FETAL MONITORING

Each time the uterus contracts during normal labor, the delivery of nutrients and oxygen to the fetus is diminished. Ordinarily the fetus possesses sufficient redundancy in its reserves of these substances that the contraction has no ill effect. However, a fetus functioning "on the edge," with depleted placental reserves, may respond to each uterine contraction with a characteristic slowing of its heart rate, technically known as a "late deceleration" when viewed on an electronic fetal heart rate monitoring printout (Fig. 2). Such late decelerations, if repetitive, are considered to be nonreassuring, possibly reflecting fetal compromise during labor. Similar changes may be seen on fetal heart rate tracings of pregnant women who are not yet in spontaneous labor but who have had contractions artificially induced with an intravenous infusion of oxytocin. The oxytocin challenge test consists of the induction of at least three uterine contractions during a 10-min epoch. If all three contractions are followed by late decelerations of the fetal heart rate, the test is considered positive and indicative of a high likelihood of fetal compromise.

In the course of the performance of thousands of records of fetal heart rate monitoring, it has been noted that the healthy fetus usually demonstrates a transient increase in its heart rate after any vigorous fetal movement. The presence of two to three such accelerations of at least 15 beats/min, lasting at least 15 s, during a 20-min period is associated with a high likelihood of fetal well-being and is called a reactive nonstress test (NST) (Fig. 3). Because the NST requires only an electronic fetal monitor and not an intravenous infusion, it is simpler to perform than the oxytocin challenge test and is often used as a primary test of fetal well-being. A reactive NST is a very strong indicator of fetal well-being, but a nonreactive NST may be seen in fetal sleep states, fetal immaturity, and other situations that are not necessarily adverse. Thus, a nonreactive NST is usually followed up by another fetoplacental function test, such as a biophysical profile.

The biophysical profile is thought to combine the evaluation of chronic and acute fetal problems. In this test, the NST is combined with an ultrasound evaluation of fetal movement, fetal tone (flexion of the extremities), amniotic fluid volume, and fetal breathing. Each category is assigned a score of 0 (bad) or 2 (good) points. A score of 8–10 is ideal, 4–6 suggests possible fetal jeopardy or asphyxia, and 0–2 is very strongly indicative of fetal compromise.

Different perinatal centers use different combinations of the above antepartum tests in the evaluation of the diabetic pregnancy. There is no single approach on which there is universal agreement. However, certain principles are generally accepted. Most centers would not start any type of antepartum testing until a gestational age at which there is a possibility of fetal survival if delivery is accomplished. Thus, there is no point in doing any of these tests at 20 wk of gestation. Because all of these tests can yield false-positive results, they should not be performed if a particular patient has little risk of fetal problems; in such patients, the predictive accuracy of a positive test is poor. Thus, a particular center might defer antepartum testing until 35 wk in a patient with well-controlled diabetes who has no vascular complications but might start at 28 wk, or even earlier in a poorly controlled patient who has nephropathy, hypertension, and a growth-retarded fetus. In addition, these tests should be performed in a center where there is adequate day-to-day experience in the performance and interpretation of whatever approach is chosen. Finally, the interval of testing may vary from once per week to daily, depending on the circumstances of a particular patient.

AMNIOCENTESIS FOR FETAL LUNG MATURITY DETERMINATION

Several early studies suggest that respiratory distress syndrome, histologically known as hyaline membrane disease, occurs with increased frequency and at later gestational ages in infants of diabetic mothers. Tissue culture experiments have linked this problem with fetal hyperinsulinemia, brought about by suboptimal

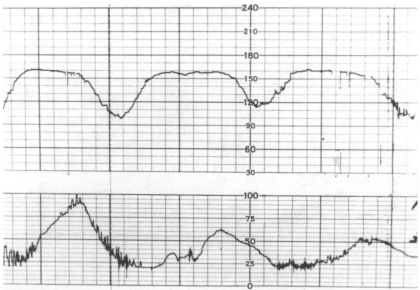

Top panel, fetal heart rate; bottom panel, uterine contractions. Note fetal heart rate dip to 100 beats/min after contraction.

Figure 2. Late Deceleration

maternal metabolic control. The use of amniotic fluid biochemical analysis can identify fetuses at greatest risk for respiratory distress syndrome if delivered and fetuses highly unlikely to develop this complication. Amniocentesis is therefore quite useful in evaluating lung maturity in the fetus of a diabetic mother. Because there were reports of a relatively high false-positive rate when the traditional lecithin-sphingomyelin ratio was used, many centers now test for the presence of phosphatidylglycerol as a highly reliable sign of lung maturity.

TIMING AND MODE OF DELIVERY

At one time, it was fairly routine to deliver infants of diabetic mothers at some arbitrary number of weeks before term to lessen the likelihood of unexplained fetal death in utero. Because of the need for early delivery when the uterine cervix was not yet "ripe" to facilitate induction of labor and because fetal macrosomia complicated a significant proportion of these pregnancies, cesarean section was the routine route of birth. The advent of antepartum testing, as described above, allowed the identification of particular pregnancies at high risk for impending intrauterine fetal death, so that the less threatened fetuses could be allowed to continue nearer to term. Most important, modern approaches to metabolic normalization of the pregnant woman with diabetes have prevented fetal deterioration, so that early delivery is less likely to be necessary. Because pregnancies allowed to progress closer to term are more likely to result in vaginal delivery and because improved metabolic control has lowered, but not eliminated, the likelihood of fetal macrosomia, most individuals with diabetes can be safely delivered vaginally.

FETAL SURVEILLANCE DURING LABOR

Because preexisting diabetes represents a high-risk situation with an increased possibility of fetal compromise, the fetal condition should be continuously evaluated with an electronic fetal monitoring device once labor has been established.

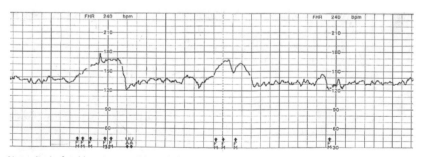

Note rise in fetal heart rate with each fetal movement (FM).

Figure 3. Fetal Monitor Strip from Nonstress Test

DIABETIC KETOACIDOSIS

An episode of diabetic ketoacidosis (DKA) carries a risk in excess of 50% for fetal death in utero. Not only is maternal acidosis dangerous for the fetus, but so is the usual dehydration that accompanies DKA. It is possible for DKA to occur in the third trimester of pregnancy with a potentially viable fetus in utero. Nonreassuring fetal heart rate tracings are very likely in such situations and can be frightening to the caregiver, because emergency cesarean section, a major surgical procedure, carries a high maternal mortality risk when performed on an individual in DKA. On the other hand, in most cases, the fetal tracing improves as the maternal DKA is corrected. For this reason, it is usually best to defer emergency cesarean section until the mother's condition has been normalized through aggressive treatment with intravenous fluids, insulin, potassium, etc. Once the mother's acid-base balance has been restored and ketosis has disappeared, the fetal heart rate tracing has usually normalized. If not, consideration can then be given to delivery for fetal indications (7–11).

PRETERM LABOR

Pregnancy in a mother with diabetes, like other pregnancies, may be complicated by preterm labor. It is arguable as to whether this complication occurs more frequently when the mother has diabetes, and there are data supportive of both points of view. Preterm labor is often treated with drugs called tocolytic agents to inhibit uterine contractions. The most common of these, ritodrine and terbutaline, have β-adrenergic agonist properties that can cause maternal hyperglycemia, hypokalemia, pulmonary edema believed to be secondary to alveolar capillary leakage, electrocardiographic abnormalities, tachycardia, and other problems. Although such agents are not absolutely contraindicated in mothers with diabetes, they should be used with extreme caution. Frequent monitoring of maternal circulating glucose levels (hourly for the first 4 h, every 2–4 h thereafter) and serum potassium, performance of an electrocardiogram before institution of these agents, and avoidance of excessive amounts of salt-containing intravenous fluids are all recommended. In mothers with type 1 diabetes, it is customary to start a constant intravenous insulin infusion at a rate ranging from 2 to 7 U/h when β-mimetic tocolytics are used parenterally. Another option is to use a nonadrenergic tocolytic agent. Intravenous magnesium sulfate is most commonly used in this situation and does not cause hyperglycemia or hypokalemia. It can cause respiratory depression when serum magnesium levels are too high, and its use has been associated with pulmonary edema in isolated cases. In summary, the mother with diabetes should not be denied tocolysis when it is indicated, but tocolytic agents should be used cautiously in such patients.

The use of corticosteroids to accelerate the process of lung maturation is commonly undertaken at <34 wk of gestation in situations where the likelihood of delivery within 1 wk is believed to be extremely high. Although the use of steroids may cause worrisome deterioration in maternal metabolic control, diabetes should not be considered an absolute contraindication. Rather, if the indication for steroid therapy is strong, such agents should be administered with attention being paid to maternal metabolism. An intravenous insulin infusion may be helpful. If steroid therapy is necessary, insulin requirements may double.

REFERENCES

1. Colman A, Maharaj D, Hutton J, Tuohy J: Reliability of ultrasound estimation of fetal weight in term singleton pregnancies. *N Z Med J* 119:U2146, 2006

2. Farrell T, Owen P, Kernaghan D, Ola B, Bruce C, Fraser R: Can ultrasound fetal biometry predict fetal hyperinsulinaemia at delivery in pregnancy complicated by maternal diabetes? *Eur J Obstet Gyncol Reprod Biol* 131:146–50, 2007

3. Chauhan SP, Parker D, Shields D, Sanderson M, Cole JH, Scardo JA: Sonographic estimate of birth weight among high-risk patients: feasibility and factors influencing accuracy. *Am J Obstet Gynecol* 195:601–06, 2006

4. Nahum GG, Stanislaw H: Accurate prediction of fetal macrosomia using combination methods. *Am J Obstet Gynecol* 195:879–80, 2006

5. Langer O: Ultrasound biometry evolves in the management of diabetes in pregnancy. *Ultrasound Obstet Gynecol* 26:585–95, 2005

6. Coomarasamy A, Connock M, Thornton J, Khan KS: Accuracy of ultrasound biometry in the prediction of macrosomia: a systematic quantitative review. *BJOG* 112:1461–66, 2005

7. Coustan DR: Diabetic Ketoacidosis: *Critical Care of the Obstetric Patient.* Berkowitz RL, Ed. New York, Churchill Livingstone, 1983, p. 411–30

8. Creasy RK, Resnick R: *Maternal-Fetal Medicine: Principles and Practice. Sect. 7. Biophysical Evaluation of the Fetus.* 3rd ed. Philadelphia, Saunders, 1994, p. 276–348

9. Jeanty P, Romero R: *Obstetrical Ultrasound.* New York, McGraw-Hill, 1984

10. Landon MB, Gabbe SG: Fetal surveillance in the pregnancy complicated by diabetes mellitus. *Clin Obstet Gynecol* 34:535–43, 1991

11. Reece EA, Coustan DR (Eds.): *Diabetes Mellitus in Pregnancy: Principles and Practice.* New York, Churchill Livingstone, 1988

Gestational Diabetes

Insulin Therapy
    Metabolic Management During Therapy
        Intensified metabolic therapy
        Goals and surveillance

Obstetric Management
    Fetal Suveillance
    Maternal Surveillance
    Timing and Route of Delivery

References

Highlights
Gestational Diabetes

■ The definition of gestational diabetes mellitus (GDM) is glucose intolerance of variable severity, with onset or first recognition during the current pregnancy. This definition applies regardless of the need for insulin or whether the diabetes disappears after the pregnancy.

■ Any woman at a very high risk of GDM (marked obesity, personal history of GDM, glycosuria, or a strong family history of diabetes) should be screened for diabetes using standard diagnostic criteria as soon as possible after confirmation of pregnancy.

■ All women of higher than low risk of GDM (see Table 24) undergo a 50-g glucose challenge test at 24–28 wk of gestation. If 1-h plasma glucose is >140 mg/dl (>7.8 mmol/l), the patient should be referred for a 3-h 100-g oral glucose tolerance test. GDM is diagnosed if two or more values are >2 SDs above the mean of the glucose tolerance test.

■ The mainstay of therapy is the dietary prescription. The goal of medical nutrition therapy (MNT) is to keep the peak postprandial glucose response in the normal range. Because the carbohydrate content of the meal is the chief component of the postprandial peak glucose level, atten-

tion must be given to limiting excess carbohydrate in meals.

■ Glucose monitoring is paramount in the gestational diabetic woman. Criteria for beginning insulin are based on the fasting and postprandial responses to the prescribed meal plan.

■ When indicated by fasting and postprandial glucose levels, therapy with human insulins is prescribed to reestablish normoglycemia.

■ Exercise programs are considered safe as an adjunct therapy for GDM.

■ Timing and mode of delivery are not only decided by the classic obstetric indications but also by the glycemic control of the mother.

■ Postpartum, insulin requirements will disappear, and in 90% of women, the diabetes will disappear. A glucose tolerance test 6–8 wk postpartum should be performed to ensure that the woman is not left with type 2 diabetes.

■ A prevention program should be started immediately postpartum to keep the woman lean and fit, which decreases the chances from 60 to 25% that she will develop type 2 diabetes as she ages.

Gestational Diabetes

Gestational diabetes mellitus (GDM) is defined as carbohydrate intolerance of variable severity with onset or first recognition during pregnancy. The definition applies regardless of whether insulin is used for treatment or the condition persists after pregnancy (1). The broad definition of GDM allows for a potentially heterogeneous group of patients. It is possible that some women with GDM may have had unrecognized diabetes, either type 1 or type 2 diabetes, antedating pregnancy (2). Because GDM is typically a disorder of late gestation, this possibility is particularly great if hyperglycemia is noted during the first trimester.

Maternal hyperglycemia and a surfeit of other metabolic fuels, i.e., plasma lipids and amino acids, increase the risk of macrosomia, birth trauma, and neonatal hypoglycemia. Furthermore, recent data indicate that the effects of GDM go well beyond the perinatal period to include long-range implications for future diabetes, obesity, and abnormal neurobehavioral development (3).

Medical care for women with GDM begins with detection. The American Diabetes Association (ADA) recommends that any pregnant women at very high risk for GDM (marked obesity, personal history of GDM, glycosuria, or a strong family history of diabetes) be screened for diabetes using standard diagnostic criteria as soon as possible after confirmation of pregnancy. For women who are not found to have diabetes in early pregnancy, and for all other pregnant women, it is recommended that all women other than those at low risk of GDM (see Table 24) should be screened for GDM at 24–28 wk of gestation. Screening generally consists of measuring plasma glucose 1 h after a 50-g oral glucose load. Women with a 1-h value of 140 mg/dl (7.8 mmol/l) or above should undergo a 3-h 100-g oral glucose tolerance test (OGTT). Diagnostic cut-points for GDM are listed in Table 27. Once the diagnosis has been established, patients should be counseled about diet, exercise, self-monitoring of blood glucose (SMBG), obstetric care, and in some cases, administration of insulin.

EPIDEMIOLOGY

The prevalence of GDM varies markedly in different parts of the world and among racial and ethnic groups within the same country. O'Sullivan and Mahan (4) reported a GDM prevalence of 2.5% in Boston, Massachusetts, whereas Mestman (5) reported a prevalence of 12.3% in Los Angeles, California, a difference likely explained by a preponderance of obese Hispanic women in the latter group. Similarly, in Australia, the prevalence of GDM differed according to country of

Table 24 Diagnosis and Management of Gestational Diabetes

Risk assessment at first prenatal visit. Immediate glucose testing for high-risk group*; screening of all pregnant women except for those in low-risk group* for gestational diabetes at 24–28 wk gestation (random 50-g 1-h oral glucose challenge)†

Plasma glucose <140 mg/dl (<7.8 mmol/l)	Plasma glucose ≥140 mg/dl (≥7.8 mmol/l)
No gestational diabetes	Administer 75-g or 100-g 3-h oral glucose tolerance test (after 8- to 14-h overnight fast and 3 days carbohydrate loading

If two or more are abnormal:
Fasting blood glucose ≥95, 1-h 180, 2-h 155, 3-h 140 mg/dl (≥5.3, 10, 8.6, 7.8 mmol/l, respectively)

Diet; monitor glycemia, fetus

Fasting blood glucose ≤95 mg/dl (≤5.8 mmol/l) and 2-h postprandial ≤120 mg/dl (≤6.7 mmol/l)	Fasting blood glucose >95 mg/dl (>5.8 mmol/l) or 2-h postprandial >120 mg/dl (6.7 mmol/l)
Continue diet; monitor glycemia and fetus	Initiate insulin treatment; monitor glycemia and fetus

From Coustan (10), with permission. Also from Ney and Hollingsworth (14).
*High-risk group: marked obesity, personal history of GDM, glycosuria, or strong family history of diabetes. Low-risk group (must meet all of the following): age <25 years, normal prepregnancy weight, member of an ethnic group with low prevalence of diabetes, no known diabetes in first-degree relative, no history of abnormal glucose tolerance, no history of poor obstetric outcome.
†The ADA's recommendation on the diagnostic criteria for GDM may change based on the International Association of Diabetes and Pregnancy Study Group (IDPSG) meeting of 2009. As of this printing, a new consensus statement had not been published.

birth, ranging from 4.3% for women born in Australia and New Zealand to 15% for women born on the Indian subcontinent (6).

In addition to population variability, the prevalence of GDM differs according to selection of testing methods and diagnostic criteria. In North America, the approach recommended by the National Diabetes Data Group (NDDG) is based on the data of O'Sullivan and Mahan (4,7) derived from a population of pregnant women. Another diagnostic approach adopted by the World Health Organization (WHO) is based on the method and criteria recommended for use in nonpregnant adults. Both approaches have been criticized because their validation lies in the subsequent risk of overt maternal diabetes rather than pregnancy outcome. With respect to GDM, the heart of the matter is the relationship between the degree of glucose intolerance and/or hyperglycemia and the risk of adverse maternal, fetal, and neonatal outcomes (8,9). Despite these controversies, participants of three international workshop-conferences on GDM supported the continued use of O'Sullivan and Mahan's criteria (see below) for the diagnosis of GDM.

Although most women with GDM return to normal glucose tolerance postpartum, the disorder is clearly associated with an increased risk of subsequent overt diabetes. Women in whom GDM was diagnosed should be educated regarding the symptoms of overt diabetes and followed postpartum at regular intervals (see page 156).

SCREENING

ADA recommends that all pregnant women with risk factors undergo screening for GDM at 24–28 wk of gestation via a 1-h 50-g oral glucose challenge, administered without regard to time of day or interval since the last meal (Table 24). If plasma glucose is >140 mg/dl (>7.8 mmol/l), a 100-g 3-h OGTT should be performed. These recommendations were endorsed by the participants of the Fourth International Workshop-Conference on Gestational Diabetes Mellitus with some clarification (7):

- A random plasma glucose measurement >200 mg/dl (>11.1 mmol/l) outside the context of a formal glucose challenge test or fasting plasma glucose >126 mg/dl (>7 mmol/l) suggests the diabetic state and warrants further investigation.
- Laboratory measurement of plasma glucose concentration is appropriately performed with enzymatic assay techniques, and current diagnostic values are based on the use of such methods. Test strips and reflectance meters are not sufficiently precise and accurate for screening and diagnosis.
- The recommendation for 1-h 50-g glucose challenge screening at 24–28 wk of gestation should not preclude earlier testing, depending on the circumstances.

Table 25 Diagnostic Criteria for Gestational Diabetes (100-g oral glucose)

Time of Test	Blood Glucose
Fasting	≥95 mg/dl (5.3 mmol/l)
1 h	≥180 mg/dl (10.0 mmol/l)
2 h	≥155 mg/dl (8.6 mmol/l)
3 h	≥140 mg/dl (7.8 mmol/l)

Two or more values must be met or exceeded. Blood glucose levels are the same for a 75-g glucose load, but there is no 3-h measurement. From ref. 13.

Note that the recommended plasma glucose threshold of 140 mg/dl (7.8 mmol/l) for further testing after the 1-h 50-g glucose challenge was arrived at by consensus. Some published data suggest that a proportion of individuals who meet the recommended criteria for GDM have screening values below this level. However, their detection requires a substantial increase in the number of full glucose tolerance tests performed.

DIAGNOSIS

A positive screening test without a confirmatory abnormal glucose tolerance test does not establish the diagnosis of GDM. The 100-g OGTT interpreted by the criteria of O'Sullivan and Mahan (4) and modified by Coustan (10) remains the most commonly used standard for the diagnosis of GDM in the United States. Alternatively, the diagnosis can be made using a 75-g glucose load, but this test is not as well validated as the 100-g OGTT. The test is performed in the morning after an overnight fast of at least 8 h but not >14 h. Although the standard recommendation is that the test should be preceded by at least 3 days of unrestricted activity and diet, there are no data to prove that the results of the OGTT are affected by this advice. In fact, the advice is counterproductive if a woman has glucose intolerance. Three days of carbohydrate loading may be harmful to the unborn child when a woman has diabetes (8). A 100-g glucose load is given in a volume of at least 400 ml fluid. Venous plasma glucose levels are measured fasting and at 1, 2, and 3 h. Definitive diagnosis requires that two or more of the threshold values be met or exceeded (Table 25). Capillary blood measurements with glucose oxidase–impregnated test strips are not sufficiently precise and accurate for diagnostic purposes. Likewise, measurement of A1C has not been shown to provide a sensitive diagnostic test for GDM, although when the laboratory has a normal range for pregnant women, then it appears that an A1C >5.3% is associated with an a positive glucose tolerance test (11).

The above-mentioned diagnostic strategy endorsed by each of the international workshop-conferences on GDM is widely used in North America (10). However, other diagnostic criteria are used throughout the world. Another approach, supported by WHO, is based on the method and criteria used in nonpregnant adults. The WHO method uses a 75-g glucose load and interposes an intermediate diagnostic category of impaired glucose tolerance between normal and GDM. Ongoing efforts are being made to achieve global acceptance of uniform diagnostic criteria. It has also been suggested that the presence of one abnormal value on a glucose tolerance test merits treatment or further evaluation because it may be associated with increased fetal morbidity (8,9). This approach is used at some medical centers in the U.S. (12).

NUTRITIONAL MANAGEMENT

Nutritional counseling is the cornerstone of the management of all women with GDM and is based on the standard nutritional recommendations for pregnant women (1,9,13). All women with GDM should receive nutritional counseling by a registered dietitian when possible. Individualization of medical nutrition therapy (MNT) depending on maternal weight and height is recommended (13). The nutrition plan is effective if it:

- Provides the necessary nutrients for maternal/fetal health
- Results in normoglycemia
- Prevents ketosis
- Results in appropriate weight gain

Women with well-controlled GDM have the same chance of delivering a healthy baby as the general pregnant population. Through the combined efforts of the health care team and the patient, dietary management of GDM may be successful in 75% of cases.

GOALS

Although normoglycemia is the accepted goal of managing the gestational diabetic woman, the means to that end remain controversial. Dietary management has been used in the treatment of pregnancies complicated by diabetes since the 19th century. Since 1898, diets prescribed for individuals with diabetes have ranged from extremely high fat (85% of calories) to undernutrition and fasting. From the early insulin years (1922–1940) to the present, the carbohydrate content of the diabetic diet has steadily risen from 35% of calories to the previously recommended level of 55–60% of calories (14). Now ADA recommends individualizing the carbohydrate content of the diet to achieve normoglycemia.

Specifically, ADA recommends that women with GDM receive nutritional recommendations based on an individual nutritional assessment (5). Dietitians base their guidelines for nutritional management on a combination of nutrient requirements in pregnancy combined with dietary management of diabetes and SMBG (8,15).

The goals of MNT in GDM are to:

- Achieve and maintain normoglycemia (8), defined as fasting plasma glucose ≤95 mg/dl (≤5.3 mmol/l), 1-h postprandial plasma glucose ≤140 mg/dl (≤7.8 mmol/l), and/or 2-h postprandial plasma glucose ≤120 mg/dl (≤6.7 mmol/l). Recent literature suggests that these limits be decreased to ≤90 mg/dl (≤5.0 mmol/l) and/or <120 mg/dl (<6.7 mmol/l) to minimize the risk of bearing a macrosomic infant (16,17).
- Provide a nutritionally adequate diet for pregnancy. A nutritionally adequate diet contains all the essential nutrients required for fetal development and maintenance of maternal health. It also provides sufficient calories for the woman to achieve an appropriate weight gain and for her to avoid ketonuria. Refer to pages 71–90 for the components of nutritional assessment and care plan development that pertain to women with pregestational diabetes and GDM. The subjects covered include patient responsibility, the nutrient requirements of pregnancy, assessing the diet and eating habits, determining the appropriate calorie level of the diet and MNT to reach glycemic and health goals, and weight-gain recommendations.

FACTORS AFFECTING BLOOD GLUCOSE LEVELS

Tight control of blood glucose levels is necessary during pregnancy because the fetus can be adversely affected by maternal hyperglycemia. The factors that affect blood glucose levels are:

- Stress (physical stress in the form of trauma, inflammation, infection, or hormonal imbalance due to growth and development, menstrual cycle, or pregnancy; exogenously administer steroids; and psychological stress)
- Time of day
- Exercise
- Amount of carbohydrate eaten

Stress, both psychological and physical, increases blood glucose levels via contrainsulin hormones, including during pregnancy. Pregnancy increases the normal morning glucose intolerance caused by high levels of cortisol, progesterone, and growth hormone (chorionic sommatomammotropin). For this reason, hyperglycemia after breakfast commonly occurs in GDM unless carbohydrate is restricted. Greater percentages of carbohydrate can be tolerated later in the day.

The time of day also affects blood glucose levels due to the diurnal variation of contrainsulin hormones. Exercise decreases blood glucose levels by increasing the uptake of glucose into the cells without extra insulin.

Carbohydrate. The amount of carbohydrate consumed in a meal or snack is highly correlated with the effect on blood glucose (18,19). The greater the percentage of carbohydrate in the meal, the higher the resultant blood glucose level. (Individual and intraindividual variability in glycemic response does exist, however, and this information is obtained by SMBG.)

In gestational diabetes, the type of carbohydrate consumed affects blood glucose levels (18,19). Processed foods containing sugars can elevate the blood glucose level quickly. They usually peak in the bloodstream 1 h after ingestion. Sugars are easily digested, have a low satiety value, and are often in liquid form. Examples of beverages and foods containing simple sugars are fruit juices, soft drinks, milk, candy, cookies, and cakes.

The total amount of carbohydrate must be counted to predict its effect on the blood glucose level. Legumes, vegetables, and some starches peak in the bloodstream after 2 h. They are not liquid, and in general, the less refined the food, the lower the glycemic response.

Fiber. Fiber is a general term for all plant material that cannot be broken down by enzymes in the human digestive tract. Different types of dietary fiber have distinctive characteristics that enable them to function differently in the body.

Soluble fibers contained in beans, fruits, and oat bran may help lower glycemic response. These fibers tend to form gels that are thought to delay the absorption of nutrients from the intestine. This slowed absorption allows for a more gradual influx of glucose into the blood, creating less of an insulin demand.

Insoluble fiber, such as wheat bran, speeds the movement of food through the gastrointestinal tract. It increases fecal bulk, reducing constipation.

Table 26 Factors Affecting Glycemic Index of Foods*

- Processing
- Preparation
- Ripeness
- Storage
- Fiber
- Other foods ingested
- Physical form
- Digestibility of the starch component

*Anatomical and pathological factors that affect the glycemic index of foods include delayed gastric emptying and/or gastroparesis, malabsorption, short bowel syndrome, gastric bypass, pancreatitis, ileus, hypoglycemia, and diabetic neuropathy, with resultant increased or decreased transit time of food through the gut.

Glycemic index. The glycemic index is defined as the percentage increase in blood glucose after ingesting a food compared with glucose. Many characteristics of the food/meal contribute to the glycemic response (Table 26). There is a great deal of individual and intra-individual variability in glycemic response based on anatomical and pathological variables as well as the amount of fat consumed with the carbohydrate. Therefore, patients must develop their own "glycemic index" by monitoring food intake and the postprandial blood glucose responses.

DIETARY GUIDELINES

Nutritional counseling is the cornerstone of the management of women with GDM (20). It is helpful to provide women with basic dietary guidelines ("dos and don'ts") *1)* to promote normoglycemia and avoid excessive weight gain and *2)* to develop an individual meal plan with the patient (Table 27). The rationale for each recommendation is briefly described below.

- **Avoid concentrated sweets.**
  Rationale: These foods cause hyperglycemia in women with GDM; they are usually high in calories and low in nutrients. Emphasize fresh foods.
- **Avoid highly processed foods.**
  Rationale: Eating highly processed foods usually results in a more rapid rise in blood glucose than fresh or less processed foods. These foods are often high in fat, contributing to excessive weight gain.
- **Eat small meals.**
  Rationale: Consuming small frequent meals helps women avoid postprandial hyperglycemia and preprandial starvation ketosis. A consistent meal pattern is important: three meals and three snacks are usually recommended. Snacks prevent women from becoming overly hungry and overeating at the next meal. Protein foods are encouraged because they are

Table 27 Dietary Guidelines for Women With Gestational Diabetes (or Those at Risk)

Avoid concentrated sweets
- No cookies, cakes, pies, soft drinks, chocolate, table sugar, fruit juices, fruit drinks, Kool-Aid, Hi-C, nectars, jams, or jellies

Avoid convenience foods
- No instant noodles, canned soups, instant potatoes, frozen meals, or packaged stuffing

Eat small frequent meals
- Eat about every 3 hours
- Include a good source of protein at every meal and snack. High-protein foods are low-fat meat, chicken, fish, low-fat cheese, nuts, peanut butter, cottage cheese, eggs, and turkey

Eat a very small breakfast
- No more than one starch exchange (<15 g carbohydrate) and thus must limit cereal (cooked or cold are equally potent and produce postprandial hyperglycemia), bread, pancakes, toast, bagels, muffins, and Danishes
- No fruit or juice

Choose high-fiber foods
- Fresh and frozen vegetables
- Beans and legumes
- Fresh fruits (except at breakfast)

Free foods—eat as desired:

cabbage	mushrooms	celery	radishes
cucumbers	zucchini	green beans	lettuce
green onions	spinach	onions and garlic	broccoli
asparagus	nopales	spinach	lemons/limes
avocado	olive oil/olives	butter	sour cream

Adapted from the Santa Barbara Diabetes Initiative–In collaboration with the Sansum Diabetes Research Institute, Santa Barbara Neighborhood Clinics, American Indian Health & Services, and Santa Barbara County Health Care Services, Nutrition Division. Funded by the California Endowment 2005–2008.

digested and absorbed more slowly than carbohydrates, yielding a lower glycemic response. The fat in protein foods contributes to a greater satiety value than carbohydrate-rich foods, preventing excessive hunger. The small frequent meal pattern also helps to alleviate nausea and heartburn, two common discomforts of pregnancy.
- **Eat a very small breakfast.**
  Rationale: A small breakfast, low in carbohydrate (<10%), is needed because morning blood glucose levels are likely to be high in patients with

GDM. Fruits and juices should be avoided; milk should be limited (or omitted if postprandial hyperglycemia results). Highly processed breakfast cereals should be excluded.

■ **Free foods (eat as desired): celery, lettuce, broccoli, cauliflower, nopales, cheese, proteins, asparagus, tomatoes, etc.**

Rationale: These foods provide <20 kcal/serving, are very low in carbohydrate, and may be eaten when patients are hungry. These foods can be prepared as soups or eaten raw as salads.

INDIVIDUALIZED MEAL PLANNING

Composition of the diet. ADA recommends that the dietary prescription be based on nutritional assessment and treatment goals. There is no standard "ADA diet." The dietary guidelines in this chapter are derived from literature review and the clinical experience and recommendations of practitioners in diabetes and pregnancy programs (18–21). Therefore, the recommended composition of the diet for women with GDM is to minimize the carbohydrate content of the meal plan and thus minimize the postprandial glucose excursions.

Within this prescription, complex carbohydrates, monounsaturated and polyunsaturated fats, and foods high in fiber are encouraged. With this attention to carbohydrate intake, normoglycemia is maintained in 75–80% of gestational diabetic women, whereas a higher carbohydrate intake results in more frequent episodes of hyperglycemia, with more women requiring insulin. If higher carbohydrate levels are prescribed, postprandial SMBG needs to be encouraged to indicate whether the diet successfully maintains postprandial blood glucose levels in the desired range (18,20).

Developing the meal plan. Distribution of calories has also been a source of controversy. Many programs recommend three meals and three snacks, regardless of whether the patient is taking insulin. Others feel that an overweight patient with GDM achieves better glucose control by simply consuming three meals and a bedtime snack (to prevent nocturnal ketone production).

Snacks can be advantageous. Protein-containing snacks between meals prevent extreme hunger at the next meal, and smaller meals and snacks every few hours are easier for pregnant women to digest.

A recommended calorie distribution to maintain normoglycemia is found in Table 28 (20). The calorie and carbohydrate levels at breakfast are quite low because of morning insulin resistance. A high-protein snack 2–3 h after breakfast is desirable to prevent excessive hunger at lunch.

The meal pattern is developed on an individual basis, based on the nutritional assessment of the patient. The diet must be consistent with the patient's lifestyle, food preferences, and cultural habits. A qualified educator, preferably a registered dietitian, should teach the patient, emphasizing appropriate portion sizes. Next, the educator should determine the appropriate calorie level and the amount of carbohydrate, protein, and fat for the individual. The educator should then record the number of servings from each food group to include in the daily diet. With the patient, the educator needs to develop a sample menu. To verify that the patient

Table 28 Calorie Distribution to Maintain Normoglycemia

Meal	Calories (%)
Breakfast	10–15
Snack	5–10
Lunch	20–30
Snack	5–10
Dinner	30–40
Snack	5–10

understands the meal plan, the patient should be asked to plan another sample menu, using a resource such as *Choose Your Foods: Plan Your Meals* or *Choose Your Foods: Exchange Lists for Meal Planning*.

CONTROVERSY: CALORIE RESTRICTION FOR OBESE PATIENTS

A recent area of interest is the use of hypocaloric diets for obese women with GDM. Studies have revealed that restricting calories by 30–33% results in reduced hyperglycemia, reduced plasma triglycerides, and no increase in ketonuria (16). Elevated fasting triglyceride concentrations in GDM are more strongly associated with infant macrosomia than are fasting or postprandial glucose concentrations (22–27). The conclusion is that moderate calorie restriction may be valuable in preventing macrosomia.

Other studies showed that calorie restriction normalized birth weights in gestational diabetic mothers with no increase in perinatal morbidity (22,23). Also, fewer women required insulin. One explanation for these results is that the women experienced an improvement in insulin sensitivity secondary to calorie restriction. The women in this study gained only 1.7 ± 1.6 kg (3.7 ± 3.5 lb) during the third trimester. Another potential advantage of calorie restriction is less postpartum obesity, which lessens the risk of future diabetes (28).

The calorie-restricted approach might decrease the concentration of all maternal fuels reaching the fetal circulation (amino acids, plasma triglyceride fatty acids, and glucose), thereby reducing macrosomia. However, levels of free fatty acids and ketones may increase, so further research is needed to determine whether calorie restriction might adversely affect the future health of the infant (1).

RECORD KEEPING AND FOLLOW-UP

The patient must be taught to keep food and blood glucose records, recording the time of the meal or snack and the amount and kinds of foods and beverages consumed. Checking blood glucose four times a day is recommended:

■ Fasting (after rising)

- 1 h after breakfast
- 1 h after lunch
- 1 h after dinner

The diet prescription must be validated with blood glucose monitoring: the diet only "fits" if no postprandial hyperglycemia results (1-h postprandial blood glucose <120 mg/dl [6.7 mmol/l]). The food records also help the dietitian to know whether the patient understands the diet. The records should be evaluated at every visit to provide vital feedback to the patient. The records are important because:

- Individual food sensitivities can be pinpointed (e.g., foods that yield a high glycemic response).
- They allow the dietitian to evaluate the patient's understanding of the meal plan and to provide appropriate continuing education.
- Perhaps most important, they help the patient learn to make decisions about what and how much to eat, putting her in control.

Prenatal nutritional supplements are often used in pregnancy, since it is difficult to assess adequacy of micronutrient intake. Iron is recommended as an additional nutritional supplement in women with iron deficiency anemia.

POSTPARTUM

Women with GDM have a 40–60% chance of developing type 2 diabetes as they age (1). It has been reported that this prevalence rate can be reduced to 25% if these women become lean and fit after delivery (28). With an appropriate weight loss and fitness program, these women can improve their health and lower their risk of developing diabetes.

Breastfeeding should be encouraged in women with GDM. There are numerous physiological and emotional advantages of breastfeeding over formula feeding. Although not all women lose weight while breastfeeding, it is normal for weight loss to occur because of a greater energy expenditure during lactation (see also page 83).

EXERCISE AS A TREATMENT MODALITY

GDM is considered to be in part a disease of glucose clearance, although it has been shown that this disorder is a heterogeneous entity (25). A treatment modality that overcomes the peripheral resistance to insulin, such as exercise, might be preferable to insulin administration. Cardiovascular conditioning exercise facilitates glucose utilization among other things by increasing insulin binding to and affinity for its receptor and receptor number (26).

Although exercise during pregnancy has been gaining acceptance (27), it remains controversial. The conclusions are that the safest form of exercise is that which does not cause fetal distress, low infant birth weight, uterine contractions, or maternal hypertension (blood pressure >140/90 mmHg) (28–31). Appropriate exercises are those that use the upper-body muscles or place little mechanical stress on the trunk region during exercise (32). When the lower body is kept from an excessive weight-bearing load, the work load can be increased safely, permitting a cardiovascular workout without fear of fetal distress. Women may be taught to palpate their own uterus during exercise and stop the exercise if they detect a contraction. In addition to proper frequency, intensity, duration, and modality of exercise, self-monitoring of uterine activity may be a means of surveillance that allows the safe prescription of exercise during the third trimester.

Upper-body cardiovascular training has resulted in lower levels of glycemia than in women treated by diet only (33). The effects of exercise on glucose metabolism can become apparent after 4 wk of training and affect both hepatic glucose output (reflected by fasting glucose levels) and glucose clearance (reflected by glucose values after a 50-g oral glucose challenge) (34). A cardiovascular conditioning program might obviate insulin treatment in some women with GDM. The Fifth International Workshop-Conference on Gestational Diabetes Mellitus advocated exercise as a treatment modality for GDM in women who do not have a medical or obstetric contraindication for an exercise program (35).

INSULIN THERAPY

Intensive management has been shown to improve infant outcome (11). However, intensive management of GDM may also provide benefit to the mothers. Rates of preterm labor, preeclampsia, maternal trauma from birth, and postpartum complications have been associated with failure to diagnose and treat GDM and with the degree of hyperglycemia in treated patients. The largest randomized controlled trial (RCT) of intensified management versus standard prenatal care of women with GDM showed less preeclampsia but a higher rate of induction of labor with intervention, as well as improved postpartum health status and less depression (36). Other RCTs provide more data on maternal benefits of treatment of GDM (37).

METABOLIC MANAGEMENT DURING PREGNANCY

A recent RCT (36) demonstrated that treating GDM (diagnosed when the 2-h value after a 75-g oral glucose load was 140–198 mg/dl [7.8–11.0 mmol/l] and mean fasting plasma glucose was 86 ± 13 mg/dl [4.8 ± 0.7 mmol/l]) significantly reduced the likelihood of serious neonatal morbidity compared with routine prenatal care. Treatment included individualized MNT, daily SMBG, and insulin when needed (20%) (36). Similar RCTs (38) have also been conducted. Based on the Australian RCT (36) as well as other lower-level data on pregnancy outcome in untreated GDM (37–41), diagnosis and management of GDM is supported, with onset of treatment by 30 wk of gestation.

Intensified metabolic therapy. To determine whether dietary management is effective in maintaining euglycemia, blood glucose concentration must be monitored regularly. The use of insulin is widely recommended when appropriate MNT does not consistently maintain normal fasting plasma glucose ≤95 mg/dl (≤5.3 mmol/l) or 2-h postprandial plasma glucose ≤120 mg/dl (≤6.7 mmol/l). To prevent macrosomia, it has been recommended that insulin be started when fasting plasma glucose is >90 mg/dl (>5.0 mmol/l) and/or 1-h postprandial glucose is >120 mg/dl

(>6.7 mmol/l) (11). An isolated glucose level can often be attributed to a temporary dietary indiscretion. However, two or more glucose measurements within 1 or 2 wk that exceed the recommended goals should prompt either the reassessment of glycemia within the next few days or the institution of insulin therapy.

To safely initiate insulin therapy, qualified educators must be available to teach the basic timing and action of insulin; proper injection technique; dietary adjustments; and recognition, avoidance, and treatment of hypoglycemia. In offices or clinics staffed with diabetes care professionals, insulin may be initiated in the outpatient setting with close and frequent contact. Without such expertise, patients should be hospitalized to begin therapy and to titrate the dosage. There are no data demonstrating superiority of a particular insulin regimen in GDM. It is recommended that insulin administration be individualized to achieve the glycemic goals stated above.

Human insulin is the least immunogenic of the commercially available preparations, but the three rapid-acting insulin analogs (lispro, aspart, and glulysine) are comparable in immunogenicity to human regular insulin. Insulin preparations of low antigenicity will minimize the transplacental transport of insulin antibodies. Of the three rapid- and short-acting insulin analogs, only lispro and aspart have been investigated in pregnancy, with acceptable safety profiles, minimal transfer across the placenta, and no evidence of teratogenesis. These two insulin analogs both improve postprandial excursions compared with human regular insulin and are associated with lower risk of delayed postprandial hypoglycemia. RCTs have not been carried out using long-acting insulin analogs in pregnancy (insulin glargine, insulin detemir) and they are category C in pregnancy. Thus, human NPH insulin as part of a multiple injection regimen should be used for longer-acting insulin effect in GDM. Research is needed on possible placental transfer of insulin analogs during labor, along with a registry to document use of insulins glulysine, glargine, and detemir in pregnancy.

Regarding oral *antihyperglycemic agents*, of the sulfonylurea drugs, only *glyburide* (glibenclamide) has been demonstrated to have minimal (4%) transfer across the human placenta and has not been associated with excess neonatal hypoglycemia in the few studies available. There is evidence from one RCT (42) during pregnancy and supporting observational studies that glyburide is a useful adjunct to MNT/physical activity regimens when additional therapy is needed to maintain target glucose levels (level A evidence). Glyburide must be carefully balanced with meals and snacks to prevent maternal hypoglycemia (as with insulin therapy). There is some evidence that glyburide may be less successful in obese patients or patients with marked hyperglycemia earlier in pregnancy. As with MNT/physical activity and insulin regimens, SMBG and fetal measurements of abdominal circumference (AC) or other parameters of fetal size need to be followed closely in women using glyburide. More research is needed to determine 1) if maternal and neonatal outcomes with glyburide are equivalent to those obtained with insulin therapy; 2) if there are glyburide effects on the potential postpartum progression of the woman with GDM toward glucose intolerance/diabetes, or on the possibility of GDM recurrence; and 3) whether there are glyburide effects on the well-being of offspring at medium and long term.

Metformin does cross the placenta, and at present, there is no evidence to recommend metformin treatment for GDM except in clinical trials, which should include long-term follow-up of infants. Metformin has been used in nonrandomized studies of women with polycystic ovary syndrome in pregnancy, but there is insufficient evidence that metformin prevents GDM.

Acarbose, an α-glucosidase inhibitor, is poorly absorbed from the gastrointestinal tract, and two preliminary studies have suggested efficacy in reducing postprandial glucose excursions in GDM, but with the expected frequency of abdominal cramping. Because a small proportion of this drug may be absorbed systemically, further study should evaluate potential transplacental passage. Use of thiazolidinediones, glinides, and glucagon-like peptide (GLP)-1 during pregnancy is considered experimental. There are no controlled data available in pregnancy, and one study reported that rosiglitazone crossed the human placenta at 10–12 wk of gestation, with fetal tissue levels measured at about half of maternal serum levels (45). With regard to GLP-1 agonists, ex vivo human placental perfusion studies detected minimal levels on the fetal side (fetal-to-maternal ratio 0.017) (43,44).

Goals and surveillance. Table 29 provides ambulatory glucose values measured in pregnant women with normal glucose tolerance (45,46) and values used as treatment targets in clinical trials in women with GDM who achieved improved perinatal outcomes in the intervention group (36,38,41,47). The large Australian RCT that compared multifaceted treatment with routine perinatal care has been mentioned (36).

The other trials also achieved satisfactory clinical outcomes, including frequency of fetal macrosomia <11%, suggesting that the treatment targets are appropriate. However, there are no data from controlled trials of lower versus higher targets or 1- versus 2-h postprandial testing to identify ideal goals for prevention of fetal risks. Evidence from observational studies suggests that when *mean* capillary glucose levels in GDM are low (<87 mg/dl [<4.8 mmol/l]), there is an increased likelihood of infants who are small for gestational age (38).

Daily SMBG using meters with memory capability appears to be superior to less frequent monitoring in the clinic for detection of glucose concentrations that may warrant intensification of therapy beyond individualized MNT. Many providers decrease the frequency of SMBG when MNT is successful in achieving goals for metabolic control; available data do not address such issues as the duration of good control sufficient to reduce the frequency of SMBG or the appropriate frequency of testing in women with GDM who are well controlled on MNT. New technologies for glucose surveillance should enable future research to determine optimal goals for metabolic control. When alternate site testing is used, consideration should be given to the lag time for changes in postprandial glucose when compared with fingerstick capillary glucose testing. Validation of the accuracy of patients' monitoring techniques is also essential.

Assessing the fetal response to maternal GDM by ultrasound measurement of fetal AC starting in the second and early third trimesters and repeated every 3–6 wk can provide useful information (in combination with maternal SMBG levels) to guide management decisions. Tighter glycemic control targets may be selected when size of the fetal abdomen is excessive, or pharmacological therapy can be added or intensified if a large AC is detected despite seemingly good glycemic control. For this approach to be effective in clinical practice, attention should be given to the accuracy of the measurements of fetal size and maternal glucose. More

Table 29 Normal Ambulatory Glucose Values in Prospective Studies of Pregnant Women With Normal Glucose Tolerance and Upper Boundary Glucose Values Used as Treatment Targets in Clinical Trials in Women With GDM

			Glucose [mg/dl (mmol/l)]		
	Type of Study	n	Fasting (mean, 0.95 confidence interval)	Premeal	Postprandial (mean, 0.95 confidence interval)
Normal ambulatory glucose					
Parretti et al. (46)	Capillary glucose meters adjusted for plasma	51	69, 57–81 (3.8, 3.2–4.5)		1-h 108, 96–120 min (6.0, 5.3–6.7)
Yogev et al. (43)	Continuous interstitial glucose monitoring	57	75, 51–99 (4.2, 2.8–5.5)		Peak 110, 68–142 min (6.1, 3.8–7.9)
Upper boundary glucose values			Upper range	Upper range	Upper range
Langer et al. (38)	Intensified SMBG, quasi-randomized	1,145 vs. 1,316	90 (5.0)		2-h <120 (6.7)
de Veciana et al. (47)	RCT, premeal vs. postprandial glucose	33 vs. 33	90 (5.0)		1-h <140 (7.8)
Langer et al. (42)	RCT, glyburide vs. insulin	201 vs. 203	90 (5.0)	95 (5.3)	2-h <120 (7.8)
Crowther et al. (36)	RCT, intensified treatment vs. prenatal care	490 vs. 510	99 (5.5)	<100 (5.6)	2-h <127 (7.1)

Improved perinatal outcomes were achieved in the intervention groups.

prospective studies are needed to assess the cost-effectiveness of this approach compared with SMBG continued throughout pregnancy. Further study should address the addition of other measures of fetal size (subcutaneous fat and head circumference–to-AC ratio) to assessment of the fetal response to maternal management (43–47).

Urine ketone testing has been recommended in GDM patients with severe hyperglycemia, weight loss during treatment, or other concerns of possible "starvation ketosis." Fingerstick blood ketone testing is available and is more representative of laboratory measurements of β-hydroxybutyrate. However, the effectiveness of ketone monitoring (either urine or blood) in improving fetal outcome has not been tested. Insufficient data are available to determine whether measurement of glycosylated hemoglobin or other circulating proteins are of value in the routine management of GDM.

Most women with GDM will not require insulin during labor because the exercise of labor uses glucose substrate at the same intensity as running a marathon (48,49). Nevertheless, it is important to continue measuring blood glucose to detect the patients who do. When induction of labor is planned, insulin and breakfast should be omitted in the morning and intravenous fluids begun. Typically, fluids consist of 5% dextrose in half-normal saline administered at a rate of 100 ml/h i.v. It is important to avoid rapid infusion of large volumes of glucose-containing solutions because maternal hyperglycemia may cause neonatal hypoglycemia immediately after delivery. Thus, if rapid intravenous hydration is necessary before use of conduction anesthesia, non–glucose-containing solutions should be used. If blood glucose concentration is >120 mg/dl (>6.7 mmol/l), short-acting insulin may be administered via infusion at a rate of 1 U/h i.v. Adjust the dosage to maintain the blood glucose level within the range of 70–120 mg/dl (3.9–6.7 mmol/l). Insulin infusion should be discontinued immediately before delivery and, in most cases, will not need to be resumed postpartum (50).

OBSTETRIC MANAGEMENT

FETAL SURVEILLANCE

Use of fetal ultrasound for detection of congenital anomalies is suggested for women with GDM who present with A1C values >7.0% or fasting plasma glucose levels >120 mg/dl (>6.7 mmol/l), because an increased risk of major congenital malformations has been reported in such pregnancies. Use of ultrasound measurements to detect fetal macrosomia as a guide to GDM treatment is considered above in the section on metabolic goals and surveillance. Decisions regarding the commencement and frequency of surveillance for fetal well-being should be influenced by the severity of maternal hyperglycemia and the presence of other adverse clinical factors such as past poor obstetrical history or coincident hypertensive disorders. At a minimum, mothers with GDM should be taught to monitor fetal movements during the last 8–10 wk of pregnancy and to report immediately any reduction in the perception of fetal movements. Data are not available to demonstrate the optimal application of more intensive fetal monitoring, or which method is superior: cardiotocography, biophysical profile, or the assessment by Doppler ultrasound of umbilical blood flow. The latter method may be considered in situations where there is poor fetal growth. It is recognized that no fetal surveillance method is always able to detect fetal compromise. Data are insufficient to determine whether surveillance beyond self-monitoring of fetal movements is indicated in women with GDM continuing to meet the targets of glycemic control with MNT/physical activity regimens and in whom fetal growth is appropriate for gestational age. The rate of intervention is low for such well-controlled GDM pregnancies.

MATERNAL SURVEILLANCE

The frequency of spontaneous preterm birth may be increased in women with untreated GDM (51). Use of corticosteroids to enhance fetal lung maturity should not be withheld because of a diagnosis of GDM, but intensified monitoring of maternal glucose levels is indicated and temporary addition or increase of insulin doses may be necessary. The risk of hypertensive disorders is also increased in women with GDM. RCTs are needed to determine the efficacy and safety of anti-hypertensive therapy in women with GDM and chronic hypertension and whether there is any long-term benefit from treatment during pregnancy. Studies of non-diabetic women with gestational hypertension suggest that treatment is not indicated during pregnancy in the absence of albuminuria or other signs of target organ damage, but studies of gestational hypertension in women with GDM are not available. Evidence was presented at the 5th International Workshop-Conference on Gestational Diabetes Mellitus stating that women with GDM are at greater risk for vascular disease than nondiabetic women. Measurement of blood pressure and urinary protein is recommended at each prenatal visit to detect the development of preeclampsia, for which standard treatment methods should be applied in women with GDM.

Assessment of maternal capillary glucose during labor is recommended to prevent maternal hyperglycemia and fetal hypoxia and neonatal hypoglycemia. Prospective studies are needed to determine the frequency of measurement and the optimal glucose levels that are associated with the best perinatal outcome.

TIMING AND ROUTE OF DELIVERY

GDM was not felt to be an indication for delivery before 38 wk of gestation in the absence of objective evidence of fetal compromise. However, some evidence indicates that delay of delivery past 38 wk can lead to an increase in the rate of large-for-gestational-age (LGA) infants without reducing the rate of cesarean deliveries. Thus, consideration may be given to delivery once patients reach 38 completed weeks of gestation. Amniocentesis for assessment of fetal lung maturity is not indicated in well-controlled patients after 37 wk of gestation who have indications for induction of labor or cesarean section as long as there is reasonable certainty about the estimation of the gestational age. Ultrasound in the first half of pregnancy is the most accurate estimator of gestational age. When delivery appears necessary for the well-being of mother or fetus, delivery should be effected without regard to lung maturity testing.

Data are not available to indicate whether or not there is greater risk of perinatal morbidity/mortality in the infants of women with well-controlled GDM if pregnancy is allowed to proceed past 40 wk of gestation. Nevertheless, it would be reasonable to intensify fetal surveillance when pregnancy is allowed to continue beyond 40 wk of gestation.

Delivery of the LGA fetus in the setting of GDM is associated with an increased risk of birth injury compared with the nondiabetic population. Strategies to reduce the risk of birth injury have included a liberal policy toward cesarean delivery when fetal overgrowth is suspected. However, no controlled trials are available to support this approach. In planning the timing and route of delivery, considerations of fetal size using clinical and ultrasound estimation of fetal weight, despite inherent inaccuracies, are frequently used by clinicians. Incorporating ultrasound measures of estimated fetal weight (EFW) or AC into decisions regarding timing and route of delivery may be associated with a lower rate of shoulder dystocia, but larger studies are needed to determine if this approach influences the rate of neonatal injury. Ultimately, the decision regarding the mode of delivery must balance the risks of potential traumatic injury to the fetus with vaginal birth versus the principally maternal risks of cesarean delivery.

REFERENCES

1. Metzger BE: Summary and recommendations of the Fifth International Workshop-Conference on Gestational Diabetes Mellitus. *Diabetes Care* 30 (Suppl. 2):197–201, 1991

2. Omori Y, Jovanovic L: Proposal for the reconsideration of the definition of gestational diabetes mellitus. *Diabetes Care* 28:1592–93, 2005

3. Silverman BL, Rizzo T, Green OC, Cho NH, Winter RJ, Ogata ES, Richards GE, Metzger BE: Long-term prospective evaluation of offspring of diabetic mothers. *Diabetes* 40 (Suppl. 2):121–25, 1991

4. O'Sullivan JB, Mahan CM: Criteria for the oral glucose tolerance test in pregnancy. *Diabetes* 13:278–85, 1964

5. Mestman JH: Outcome of diabetes screening in pregnancy and perinatal morbidity in infants of mothers with mild impairment in glucose tolerance. *Diabetes Care* 3:447–52, 1980

6. Beischer NA, Oats JN, Henry OA, Sheedy MT, Walstab JE: Incidence and severity of gestational diabetes mellitus according to country of birth in women living in Australia. *Diabetes* 40 (Suppl. 2):35–38, 1991

7. Metzger BE, Coustan DR (Eds): Summary and recommendations of the Fourth International Workshop-Conference on Gestational Diabetes Mellitus. *Diabetes Care* 21 (Suppl. 2):B161–67, 1998

8. Jovanovic L, Pettitt, DJ: Contempo Updates: Linking evidence and experience: gestational diabetes mellitus. *JAMA* 286:2516–18, 2001

9. Pettitt DJ, Jovanovic L: Do we know how to find gestational diabetes mellitus? (Editorial) *Clin Chem* 52:1633–34, 2006

10. Coustan DR: Gestational diabetes mellitus. In *Therapy for Diabetes Mellitus and Related Disorders*. 2nd ed. Lebovitz HE, Ed. Alexandria, VA, American Diabetes Association, 1998, p. 20–26

11. Jovanovic L, Bevier W, Peterson CM: The Santa Barbara County Health Care Services Program: Birth weight change concomitant with screening for and treatment of glucose-intolerance of pregnancy: a potential cost-effective intervention. *Am J Perinatol* 14:221–28, 1997

12. Langer O, Anyaegbunam A, Brustman L, Divon MY: A prospective randomized study: management of women with one abnormal oral glucose tolerance

test value reduces adverse outcome in pregnancy. *Am J Obstet Gynecol* 161:593–99, 1989

13. American Diabetes Association: Gestational diabetes mellitus (Position Statement). *Diabetes Care* 27 (Suppl. 1):S88–90, 2004

14. Ney D, Hollingsworth DR: Nutritional management of pregnancy complicated by diabetes: historical perspective. *Diabetes Care* 4:647–55, 1981

15. American Diabetes Association: Gestational diabetes mellitus (Position Statement). *Diabetes Care* 27 (Suppl. 1):S88–90, 2004

16. State of California, Department of Health Services, Maternal and Child Health Branch: *Sweet Success: California Diabetes and Pregnancy Program Guidelines for Care.* Sacramento, CA, State Printing Office, 2007

17. Chung JH, Voss KJ, Caughey AB, Wing DA, Henderson EJ, Major CA: Role of patient education level in predicting macrosomia among women with gestational diabetes mellitus. *J Perinatol* 26:328–32, 2006

18. Peterson CM, Jovanovic-Peterson L: Percentage of carbohydrate and glycemic response to breakfast, lunch, and dinner in women with gestational diabetes. *Diabetes* 40 (Suppl. 2):172–74, 1991

19. Major CA, Henry MJ, De Veciana M, Morgan MA: The effects of carbohydrate restriction in patients with diet-controlled gestational diabetes. *Obstet Gynecol* 91:600–04, 1998

20. Jovanovic-Peterson L, Sparks SP, Peterson CM: Dietary manipulation as a primary treatment strategy for pregnancies complicated by gestational diabetes. *J Am Coll Nutr* 9:320–25, 1990

21. Franz MJ, Bantle JP, Beebe CA, Brunzell JD, Chiasson JL, Garg A, Holzmeister LA, Hoogwerf B, Mayer-Davis E, Mooradian AD, Purnell JQ, Wheeler M: Evidence-based nutrition principles and recommendations for the treatment and prevention of diabetes and related complications. *Diabetes Care* 25:148-98, 2002

22. Knopp RH, Magee MS, Raisys V, Benedetti T: Metabolic effects of hypocaloric diets in management of gestational diabetes. *Diabetes* 40 (Suppl. 2):165–171, 1991

23. Dornhorst A, Nicholls JSD, Probst F, Paterson CM, Hollier KL, Elkeles RS, Beard RW: Calorie restriction for treatment of gestational diabetes. *Diabetes* 40 (Suppl. 2):161–64, 1991

24. Jovanovic-Peterson L, Peterson CM, Reed G, NICHD-DIEP: Maternal postprandial glucose levels predict birthweight. *Am J Obstet Gynecol* 164:103–11, 1991

25. Freinkel N, Metzger BE, Phelps RL, Dooley SC, Ogata ES, Radvany RM, Belton A: Gestational diabetes mellitus: heterogeneity of maternal age, weight, insulin secretion, HLA antigens, and islet cell antibodies and the impact of maternal metabolism on pancreatic b-cell somatic development in the offspring. *Diabetes* 34 (Suppl. 2):1–7, 1985

26. Pederson O, Beck-Nielsen H, Heding L: Increased insulin receptors after exercise in patients with insulin-dependent diabetes mellitus. *N Engl J Med* 302:886–92, 1980

27. American College of Obstetricians and Gynecologists: Home Exercise Programs. Washington, DC, *Am Coll Obstet Gynecol*, May 1986

28. Artal R, Romen Y, Wiswell R: Fetal bradycardia induced by maternal exercise. *Lancet* 2:258–60, 1984

29. Pomerance JJ, Gluck L, Lynch VA: Maternal exercise as a screening test for uteroplacental insufficiency. *Obstet Gynecol* 44:383–87, 1974

30. Jovanovic L, Kessler A, Peterson CM: Human maternal and fetal response to graded exercise. *J Appl Physiol* 58:1719–22, 1985

31. Collings C, Curet LB: Fetal heart rate response to maternal exercise. *Am J Obstet Gynecol* 151:498–501, 1985

32. Durak EP, Jovanovic-Peterson L, Peterson CM: Comparative evaluation of uterine response to exercise on five aerobic machines. *Am J Obstet Gynecol* 162:754–56, 1990

33. Jovanovic-Peterson L, Peterson CM: Dietary manipulation as a primary treatment strategy for pregnancies complicated by diabetes. *J Am Coll Nutr* 9:320–25, 1990

34. Jovanovic-Peterson L, Durak EP, Peterson CM: Randomized trial of diet versus diet plus cardiovascular conditioning on glucose levels in gestational diabetes. *Am J Obstet Gynecol* 161:415–19, 1989

35. Jovanovic-Peterson L, Peterson CM: Is exercise safe or useful for gestational diabetic women? *Diabetes* 40 (Suppl. 2):179–81, 1991

36. Crowther CA, Hiller JE, Moss JR, McPhee AJ, Jeffries WJ, Robinson JS, for the Australian Carbohydrate Intolerance Study in Pregnant Women (ACHOIS) Trial Group: Effect of treatment of gestational diabetes mellitus on pregnancy outcomes. *N Engl J Med* 352:2477-86, 2005

37. Sermer M, Naylor D, Gare DJ, Kenshole AB, Ritchie JWK, Farine D, Cohen HR, McArthur K, Holzapfel S, Biringer A, Chen E, for the Toronto Tri-Hospital Gestational Diabetes Investigators: Impact of increasing carbohydrate intolerance on maternal-fetal outcomes in 3637 women without gestational diabetes: The Toronto Tri-Hospital Gestational Diabetes Project. *Am J Obstet Gynecol* 173:146–56, 1995

38. Langer O, Rodriguez DA, Xenakis EMJ, McFarland MB, Berkus MD, Arredondo F: Intensified versus conventional management of gestational diabetes. *Am J Obstet Gynecol* 170:1036–47, 1994

39. Adams KM, Li H, Nelson RL, Ogburn PL, Danilenko-Dixon DR: Sequelae of unrecognized gestational diabetes. *Am J Obstet Gynecol* 178:1321–32, 1998

40. Ostlund I, Hanson U, Bjorklund A, Hjertberg R, Eva N, Nordlander E, Swahn ML, Wager J: Maternal and fetal outcomes if gestational impaired glucose intolerance is not treated. *Diabetes Care* 26:2107–11, 2003

41. Langer O, Yogev Y, Most O, Xenakis EMJ: Gestational diabetes: the consequences of not treating. *Am J Obstet Gynecol* 192:989–97, 2005

42. Langer O, Conway DL, Berkus MD, Xenakis EM, Gonzales O: A comparison of glyburide and insulin in women with gestational diabetes mellitus. *N Engl J Med* 343:1134–38, 2000

43. Yogev Y, Ben-Haroush A, Chen R, Rosenn B, Hod M, Langer O: Diurnal glycemic profile in obese and normal weight nondiabetic pregnant women. *Am J Obstet Gynecol* 191:949–53, 2004

44. Hiles RA, Bawdon RE, Petrella EM: Ex vivo human placental transfer of the peptides pramlintide and exentide. *Hum Exp Toxicol* 22:623–28, 2003

45. Chan LY, Yeung JH, Lau TK: Placental transfer of rosiglitazone in the first trimester of human pregnancy. *Fertil Steril* 83:955–58, 2005

46. Parretti E, Meccaci F, Papini M, Cioni R, Carignani L, Mignosa M, La Torre P, Mello G: Third-trimester maternal blood glucose levels from diurnal profiles in nondiabetic pregnancies: correlation with sonographic parameters of fetal growth. *Diabetes Care* 24:1319–23, 2001

47. de Veciana M, Major CA, Morgan MA, Asrat T, Toohey JS, Lien JM, Evans AT: Postprandial versus preprandial blood glucose monitoring in women with gestational diabetes mellitus requiring insulin therapy. *N Engl J Med* 333:1237–41, 1995

48. American College of Obstetrics and Gynecology: Exercise during pregnancy and the post partum period: Committee Opinion No. 267. *Obstet Gynecol* 99:171–73, 2002

49 Davies GAL, Wolfe LA, Mottola MF, MacKinnon C, SOGC Clinical Practice Obstetrics Committee, Canadian Society for Exercise Physiology Board of Directors: Exercise in pregnancy and the postpartum period. *J Obstet Gynecol Can* 25:516–29, 2003

50. Jovanovic L: Glucose and insulin requirements during labor and delivery: the case for normoglycemia in pregnancies complicated by diabetes. *Endocr Pract* 10:40–45, 2004

51. Yogev Y, Langer O: Spontaneous delivery and gestational diabetes: the impact of glycemic control. *Arch Gynecol Obstet* 276:361–65, 2007

Neonatal Care of Infants of Diabetic Mothers

Highlights
Neonatal Care of Infants of
Diabetic Mothers

■ Although many infants of diabetic mothers (IDMs) have an uneventful perinatal course, there is still an increased rate of complications.

■ Of factors influencing neonatal morbidity in diabetic pregnancies, the most significant single factor is the gestational age of the pregnancy.

■ Maintenance of a normal metabolic state, including euglycemia, should diminish but will not eradicate the increased potential for perinatal and neonatal morbidities.

■ IDMs should optimally be delivered in tertiary care centers where there is specialized management.

■ Resuscitation requires a fully equipped area and knowledgeable personnel. Evaluation of the IDM should include observation for macrosomia, birth injury, avoidance of asphyxia, presence of congenital malformations, respiratory distress, and hypoglycemia.

■ Nursery care of the infant can be accomplished in a regular nursery or special care unit if one exists in the delivery hospital. The more appropriate the weight relative to the gestational age of the infant, the greater chance for care in a regular nursery.

Neonatal Care of Infants of Diabetic Mothers

The infant of the diabetic mother (IDM) is an excellent example of the morbidities that may exist in the neonate because of maternal disease (1). Developmentally, the normal neonate is in a transitional state of glucose homeostasis. The fetus is completely dependent on his or her mother for glucose transfer in utero, and maintenance of glucose homeostasis may be a significant problem. The neonate must maintain a balance between glucose deficiency and excess. The dependence of the conceptus on the mother for continuous substrate delivery contrasts with the variable and intermittent exogenous oral intake by the neonate. Development of homeostasis results from a balance between substrate availability and developmental hormonal, sympathomimetic, and enzymatic systems (2). The precarious nature of this balance is reinforced by the numerous morbidities producing or associated with altered states of neonatal glucose homeostasis (see page 6).

Although many IDMs have an uneventful perinatal course, there is still an increased risk of complications, even in the infant born to a woman with gestational diabetes. This section highlights specific factors that are important in the immediate care of the IDM in the delivery room, in the nursery, and subsequently after discharge from the hospital. The IDM has been the subject of extensive reviews (1–7).

PERINATAL MORTALITY AND MORBIDITY

The physician responsible for the care and delivery of the mother must inform the physician responsible for the care of the neonate well in advance of delivery. Factors of importance include:

- Knowledge of the character of the maternal diabetes (including diabetes type and degree of glucose and blood pressure control)
- Prior pregnancy history
- Complications occurring during the pregnancy (including results of fetal monitoring for evaluation of fetal size and maturity, episodes of maternal infection, vaginal bleeding, and medications administered)

Knowing these facts allows the physician caring for the neonate to anticipate many of the potential fetal and neonatal complications. These factors determine that a neonatologist be present at delivery.

Although some have concluded that peripheral hospitals away from a centralized facility should only offer to manage pregnant type 1 diabetic women if they have an antenatal/endocrine unit and a neonatal intensive care unit (8,9), all pregnant diabetic women may not be able to be transferred to a centralized facility for care. However, the physicians caring for the mother and for the neonate must foresee any complications that may arise.

Hanson et al. (10) evaluated factors influencing neonatal morbidity in diabetic pregnancies. In 92 consecutive pregnancies, those with severe morbidity had:

- Longer duration of maternal diabetes
- Shorter gestational age at birth
- Higher rates of cesarean section
- Higher frequency of preeclampsia

The most significant single factor was the gestational age of the pregnancy. Glucose control between 70 and 153 mg/dl (3.8 and 8.5 mmol/l) did not influence morbidity. Thus, the maintenance of a normal metabolic state including euglycemia should diminish, but will not completely eradicate, the increased perinatal and neonatal mortality and morbidities of diabetic pregnancy.

More recently, the role of maternal hyperglycemia and the impact on neonatal outcome has been reported by Stenhouse et al. (11). They showed that neonates were ~48 g heavier at birth for each 18 mg/dl increase in maternal glycemia in 4,681 pregnancies. With the increase in birth weight, there was also an increased risk of complications in the neonatal period. Maternal diabetes still remains as the major independent risk factor for fetal macrosomia (12–17). Rates of congenital anomalies are still 8–10 times higher in the infant of the diabetic mother than the rates in infants born to nondiabetic women, and these rates have not changed over the past 20 years (11). Thus, the neonatologist must be aware that the newborn of a diabetic woman should be treated as high risk until proven otherwise.

RESUSCITATION

As with any neonate who is considered high risk, immediately after delivery, the IDM requiring resuscitation and stabilization should be taken care of in a designated resuscitation area. As noted by the *Guidelines for Perinatal Care* (17), resuscitation should be carried out in a fully equipped area illuminated to at least 100 foot-candles and containing equipment required for skilled resuscitation (Table 30). A more detailed accounting can be obtained from the guidelines. Likewise, specific personnel should be available, dedicated to devoting their complete attention to the neonate. The American Heart Association and American Academy of Pediatrics have produced materials for teaching resuscitation skills (17,18). All neonates need to be dried off initially to maintain as close to a neutral thermal environment as possible. Evaluation of the IDM in the resuscitation room requires observation for multiple factors (Table 31).

MACROSOMIA, BIRTH INJURY, AND ASPHYXIA

The neonate of the poorly controlled diabetic patient often will appear macrosomic (>4 kg [>8 lb, 13 oz] at term or >90th percentile in weight for gestational age [15]) in contrast to neonates born to the well-controlled diabetic and the non-

---

Table 30 Equipment Required in Resuscitation

- An overhead source of radiant heat that can be regulated relative to the neonate's body temperature
- Table with equipment (laryngoscope, endotracheal tube, etc.)
- Trays with medications (glucose, epinephrine, calcium)
- Oxygen, compressed air, and suction dedicated to the neonate
- Wall clock
- Charting surface
- Catheters, needles, stopcocks, infusion pumps

---

diabetic nonobese mother (1). A consequence of undetected fetal macrosomia may be a difficult vaginal delivery because of shoulder dystocia with resultant birth injury and/or asphyxia (Table 32).

Injury to the brachial plexus may appear with a variety of presentations because the nerves of the brachial plexus may be damaged. In addition to the obvious injury to the nerves of the arm, diaphragmatic paralysis occurs if the phrenic nerve is affected. Because of the associated organomegaly in the IDM, hemorrhage in the abdominal organs is possible, specifically in the liver and adrenal glands. Hemorrhage in the external genitalia of these large neonates has been noted.

Because the neonates are at high risk, intrapartum monitoring is essential to minimize potential complications. At delivery, the nursing personnel evaluating the neonate must assign Apgar scores at 1 and 5 min to document the presence or absence of asphyxia. Although the specific etiology of asphyxia is unclear, it may be caused by difficulty in the intrapartum period because of relative macrosomia. A cord pH provides early biochemical assessment of the fetus.

Asphyxia may have diverse consequences. It may affect respiratory, renal, and central nervous system (CNS) functions acutely. Thus, decreased fluid intake is usually recommended until the degree of injury to the kidneys and CNS can be determined. An important complication of asphyxia in the neonate may be later respiratory difficulties.

CONGENITAL ANOMALIES

Although most of the morbidity and mortality data for the IDM have shown improvement with advances in the care of the mothers during pregnancy, congenital anomalies remain a major unresolved problem. The three- to eightfold

---

**Table 31 Required Observation Checklist for Infants
of Diabetic Mothers in the Resuscitation Room**

■ Asphyxia	■ Hypoglycemia
■ Birth injury	■ Tetany
■ Congenital malformations	■ Erythremia
■ Evidence of macrosomia	■ Respiratory distress

Table 32 Potential Birth Injuries in Infants of Diabetic Mothers

- Abdominal organ injury
- Brachial plexus injuries
- Cephalohematoma
- Clavicular fracture
- Diaphragmatic paralysis

- External genitalia hemorrhage
- Facial palsy
- Ocular hemorrhage
- Subdural hemorrhage

increase in the incidence of congenital anomalies in the IDM has been long noted in most centers and remains a frequent contributor to perinatal mortality (19–25; Table 33).

The pathogenesis of the increased frequency of congenital anomalies among the IDMs remains obscure (16). Several etiologies have been proposed to account for the incidence of anomalies:

- Hyperglycemia, either preconceptional or postconceptional
- Hypoglycemia
- Uteroplacental vascular disease
- Genetic predisposition

Although there are data to support each proposal, the evidence is best for the preconceptional and early postconceptional hyperglycemia etiology (19–25). The critical period of teratogenesis occurs before the seventh week postconception.

Cardiomyopathy in the IDM can be congestive or hypertrophic. Hypertrophic cardiomyopathy in neonates has been associated with poorly controlled diabetes in the mother and neonatal hypoglycemia. Respiratory distress can be accompanied by septal hypertrophy (26), with resolution of symptoms within 2–4 wk and of the hypertrophy within 2–12 mo (28). Hypertrophy of the interventricular septum and walls of the right and left ventricles has also been documented (29). Profound hypoglycemia after birth, consistent with the metabolic effects of neonatal hyperinsulinism, has been strongly associated with septal hypertrophy (25). Fetal hyperinsulinism may contribute directly to septal hypertrophy.

Although cardiac hypertrophy, apart from congenital heart disease, has been recognized in autopsies of IDMs for the past three decades, only within the last decade has attention been directed to a peculiar form of subaortic stenosis similar to the idiopathic hypertrophic subaortic stenosis found in adults (30). This particular entity may be associated with symptomatic congestive heart failure. As with the adult variant, in these neonates, therapy with digoxin is contraindicated because

Table 33 Discrete Patterns of Congenital Malformations in Infants of Diabetic Mothers

- Major congenital heart disease
- Musculoskeletal deformities, including caudal regression syndrome
- CNS deformities (anencephaly, spina bifida, hydrocephalus)

the resultant increased myocardial contractility has been reported to be deleterious. Propranolol appears to be the therapeutic drug of choice. Clinically, this disorder resolves spontaneously over a period of weeks to months with correction of the echocardiographic features as well.

RESPIRATORY DISTRESS

Respiratory distress, including respiratory distress syndrome (RDS), is a frequent and potentially severe complication in the IDM, although the trend toward delivering diabetic patients later rather than earlier in gestation (assisted by improvement in the assessment of fetal well-being) is lowering the incidence. Neonatal RDS (pathological correlate: hyaline membrane disease) develops because of lung immaturity in the neonate and remains a major cause of mortality. The relative risk of RDS in the IDM ≤38 wk gestational age was once reported to be more than five times higher than in neonates of nondiabetic mothers (31). Other causes of respiratory distress in the IDM exist as well (Table 34).

RDS has a typical course that is manifest by increasing oxygen requirements due to progressive respiratory compromise. Tachypnea, intercostal and subcostal retractions, nasal flaring, and expiratory grunting appearing in the first few minutes to hours of life are the cardinal signs of the disease. In uncomplicated cases, the disease usually peaks by 72 h of age. Complications commonly associated with the disease include the presence of a persistent patent ductus arteriosus in the very small (<1.5-kg [<3.3-lb]) neonate and bronchopulmonary dysplasia in neonates requiring prolonged ventilatory support and high ambient oxygen concentrations. Both of these conditions may significantly lengthen the clinical course of an otherwise self-limited disease.

RDS must be managed with particular attention to:

- Fluid administration
- Oxygen
- Correction of acidosis
- Ventilator support when necessary

To date, there have been no controlled trials of administration of exogenous surfactant to IDMs who were delivered with RDS. This therapy is being utilized clinically for treatment of RDS in the premature neonate in many centers around the country. The potential for a severely compromised neonate with respiratory difficulty of any sort would be diminished by close prenatal evaluation of surfactant sufficiency (lecithin/sphingomyelin [L/S] ratio and the presence of phosphatidyl

Table 34 Causes of Respiratory Distress in Infants of Diabetic Mothers Other Than Respiratory Distress Syndrome

■ Cardiac disease	■ Pneumomediastinum
■ Diaphragmatic hernia	■ Pneumothorax
■ Meconium aspiration	■ Transient tachypnea

glycerol), as well as meticulous resuscitative efforts.

HYPOGLYCEMIA

A rapid decrease in plasma glucose concentration after delivery is characteristic of the IDM. Values <35 mg/dl (<1.7 mmol/l) at term are abnormal and may occur within 30 min after clamping the umbilical vessels (32). Factors that influence the degree of hypoglycemia include previous maternal glucose homeostasis and maternal glycemia during delivery (2). An inadequately controlled pregnant diabetic woman will have stimulated the fetal pancreas to synthesize excessive insulin, which may be readily released. Administration of intravenous dextrose during the intrapartum period, which results in maternal hyperglycemia >125 mg/dl (>6.9 mmol/l), will be reflected in the fetus and will exaggerate the neonate's normal postdelivery fall in plasma glucose concentration. Hypoglycemia may persist for 48 h or may develop after 24 h (33).

The neonate exhibits transitional control of glucose metabolism, which suggests that a multiplicity of factors affect homeostasis. Many of the factors are similar to those that influence homeostasis in the adult. However, there is blunted splanchnic (hepatic) responsiveness to insulin in both the preterm and term neonate compared with the adult (34). What has not been studied in the IDM are the many contrainsulin hormones that influence metabolism (33–35). If insulin is the primary glucoregulatory hormone, then contrainsulin hormones assist in balancing the effect of insulin and other factors.

NURSERY CARE

The presence of the specific morbidities discussed above requires specialized care by individuals who have the knowledge, training, and experience to handle subsequent care and follow-up. Given this consideration, the clinician should decide whether to observe the IDM in a special-care nursery or follow the neonate in the regular nursery, assuming both exist in the delivering hospital, or transfer the infant to a special-care unit at another health center (Table 35). Even if the IDM can be cared for in the regular nursery, specific metabolic abnormalities should be looked for, including:

- Hypoglycemia
- Hypocalcemia
- Hypomagnesemia
- Erythremia
- Hyperbilirubinemia

GLUCOSE HOMEOSTASIS

Relative to glucose metabolism, the IDM is a prime example of the potential of glucose disequilibrium in the neonate. Because of the transitional nature of glucose homeostasis in the newborn period in general, accentuation of disequilibrium may be enhanced in the IDM, secondary to metabolic alterations in the mother. Preventive therapy should include rigid control of maternal blood glucose

Table 35 Factors Suggesting That the Infant of a Diabetic Mother Will Need Care in a Special Care Nursery

■ Asphyxia	■ Hypoglycemia
■ Birth injury	■ Tetany
■ Congenital malformations	■ Large or small for gestational age
■ History of maternal insulin administration	

levels during pregnancy and delivery.

Plasma glucose concentrations should be obtained at delivery from the umbilical cord. IDMs can appear asymptomatic even with a relatively low plasma glucose concentration. This may be due to the initial brain stores of glycogen; however, the exact biochemistry is as yet undefined.

The use of various glucose strips and meters in the neonate have been called into question. Specific chemical determination by a glucose analyzer is indicated. This is especially true if a glucose reflectance meter is used: evaluations of glucose reflectance meters indicate they should not be used with the capillary heel-stick blood because they are neither accurate nor reliable (33,36,37).

IDMs may require parenteral treatment for maintenance of carbohydrate homeostasis. Early administration of oral feeding at <3–4 h of age may be beneficial to maintain plasma glucose concentrations that are not depressed.

The neonate who has a glucose concentration <40 mg/dl (<2.2 mmol/l) at ≤4 h of age (for both the term and preterm neonate) should be treated with glucose administered intravenously (34; Table 36). Bolus injection without subsequent infusion will only exaggerate the hypoglycemia by a rebound mechanism and is contraindicated. Once plasma glucose stabilizes to >45 mg/dl (>2.5 mmol/l), the infusion may be slowly decreased while oral feedings are initiated and advanced. If symptomatic hypoglycemia persists, higher glucose rates of ≥8–12 mg/kg min (3.6–5.5 mg/lb min) may be necessary. Because most neonates are asymptomatic, glucagon administration to prevent hypoglycemia after delivery does not appear warranted. Furthermore, glucagon may stimulate insulin release, which may exaggerate the tendency for hypoglycemia.

Prompt recognition and treatment of the hypoglycemic neonate has minimized sequelae. No specific late CNS complications have been attributed to neonatal hypoglycemia per se in the IDM (35–39).

Ultimately, the neonate will require full supplementation orally. Although proprietary formula is available, there is no contraindication to breastfeeding by the mother who is metabolically stable.

Table 36 Signs and Symptoms of Neonatal Hypoglycemia

■ Abnormal cry	■ Convulsions	■ Jitteriness
■ Apathy	■ Cyanosis	■ Lethargy
■ Apnea	■ Hypothermia	■ Tremors
■ Cardiac arrest	■ Hypotonia	■ Tachypnea

HYPOCALCEMIA AND HYPOMAGNESEMIA

Besides hypoglycemia, hypocalcemia <7 mg/dl (<0.39 mmol/l) ranks as one of the major metabolic derangements observed in the IDM (40). Serum calcium is elevated after a rise in parathyroid hormone (PTH) levels by three mechanisms:

■ Mobilization of bone calcium
■ Reabsorption of calcium in the kidney
■ Increased absorption of calcium in the intestine through action of vitamin D

In contrast, serum calcium is decreased after a rise in calcitonin, which antagonizes the action of PTH. Serum calcium may be elevated by vitamin D (1,25-di-hydroxyvitamin D), which improves absorption of calcium in the intestine after feeding and reabsorption from bone.

During pregnancy, calcium is transferred from mother to fetus concomitant with an increasing hyperparathyroid state in the mother. Calcium concentrations are higher in the fetus than in the mother. This hyperparathyroid state functions as a homeostatic compensation to restore the maternal calcium that is diverted to the fetus. Neither calcitonin nor PTH crosses the placenta.

At birth, because of the levels of calcitonin and 1,25-dihydroxyvitamin D, serum calcium falls, subsequent to interruption of maternal-fetal calcium transfer. Elevations in PTH and 1,25-dihydroxyvitamin D as early as 24 h of age ensure correction of the low serum calcium concentration.

Approximately 50% of the neonates born to type 1 diabetic women develop hypocalcemia during the first 3 days of life (41). Evaluation of the mechanisms has failed to establish prematurity or asphyxia per se as associated factors. However, the frequency and severity of serum hypocalcemia is directly related to the severity of the diabetes and is potentiated if birth asphyxia is superimposed on the clinical state. It has been postulated that the mechanism at least partially responsible for hypocalcemia is hyperphosphatemia, which is present during the initial 48 h after birth.

In the IDM, a failure of an appropriate rise in PTH concentration in response to hypocalcemia has been reported, in contrast to infants of both mothers with gestational diabetes or nondiabetic mothers. The PTH response in the normal neonate, which occurs on the second or third day, does not occur in the IDM until 48 h or later on the third or fourth day. There is some evidence that maternal diabetes may be related to suppressed neonatal parathyroid function (42).

Hypomagnesemia (<1.5 mg/dl) has been found in as many as 33% of IDMs. As with hypocalcemia, the frequency and severity of clinical symptoms are correlated with maternal status. Neonatal magnesium concentration has been correlated with that in the mother as well as with the maternal insulin requirements and concentration of intravenous glucose administered to the neonate (42). Hypocalcemia in the IDM may be secondary to decreased hypoparathyroid function as a result of the hypomagnesemia. Hypocalcemia and hypomagnesemia, which have clinical manifestations similar to those of hypoglycemia, must be considered and treated appropriately (Table 37). The long-term potential deleterious effects of either hypocalcemia or hypomagnesemia are unknown.

HYPERBILIRUBINEMIA AND ERYTHREMIA

Hyperbilirubinemia is observed more frequently in the IDM than in the normal neonate. The pathogenesis remains uncertain (1,3,4). Prematurity (biochemical immaturity) has been rejected as an explanation (43). Other etiologies of the hyperbilirubinemia have been related to hemolysis with decreased erythrocyte survival. Erythrocyte life span, osmotic fragility, and deformability have not been found to be appreciably different in IDMs who are at risk for hyperbilirubinemia (44). However, delayed clearance of the bilirubin load, measured by pulmonary excretion of carbon monoxide as an index of bilirubin production, may be a factor (39–45).

The erythremia (polycythemia is a misnomer, because only the erythrocyte mass is elevated, not the leukocyte count or the platelet count) frequently observed in IDMs may be the most important factor associated with hyperbilirubinemia. Venous hematocrits ≥65–70% have been observed in 20–40% of IDMs during the first days of life and sometimes have been associated with signs and symptoms of neonatal erythremia, such as jitteriness, seizures, tachypnea, priapism, and oliguria. Therapy with the use of a partial-exchange transfusion (10–15% of total blood volume) through the umbilical vein with plasmanate or 5% albumin has been associated with a rapid resolution of symptoms.

LONG-TERM FOLLOW-UP

What are the long-term effects of maternal diabetes on growth, development, and psychosocial and intellectual capabilities and the risk to the neonate of subsequently developing diabetes?

An early prospective study of growth and development of the IDM suggested

---

Table 37 Initial Treatment of Documented Hypoglycemia, Hypocalcemia, and Hypomagnesemia in Infants of Diabetic Mothers

Symptomatic hypoglycemia*
■ Minibolus infusion of 2 ml/kg (0.9 ml/lb) 10% dextrose in water, followed by
■ Continuous infusion of dextrose at 8 mg/kg/min (3.6 mg/lb/min)

Symptomatic hypocalcemia
■ Infusion of 1–2 ml/kg (0.5–1.0 mg/lb) 10% calcium gluconate (9–18 mg/kg [4.1–8.2 mg/lb] elemental calcium) over 5–10 min
■ Monitor heart rate
■ Maintenance therapy may be given parenterally or orally at 2–8 ml/kg/day (0.9–3.6 ml/lb/day)

Symtomatic hypomagnesemia
■ Infusion or intramuscular injection of 0.1–0.2 ml/kg (0.05–0.09 ml/lb) 50% solution (4 mEq Mg/ml)
■ Monitor heart rate
■ Repeat every 6–12 h

*From ref. 37.

that excessive weight is almost 10 times more common in children of diabetic mothers than unusually low weight, which may represent a potential "return to obesity" noted at birth in this group of neonates (46). A more recent study found that neonates >4 kg (>8 lb, 13 oz) had significant elevations of height or weight at the time of entrance to school (47). Vohr et al. (48) suggested that macrosomia in the IDM may be a predisposing factor for later obesity, because at 7 yr of age, 8 of 19 IDMs who had been large for gestational age at birth were obese, whereas only 1 of 14 who had been appropriate for gestational age was obese. When body weight and length and head circumference were evaluated from birth through 48 mo of age, children of mothers with poor control during pregnancy showed higher values for weight and the weight-to-height ratio in infancy compared with neonates of well-controlled mothers (49). Studies have shown that the offspring of a woman with GDM is at increased risk for developing obesity during adolescence and glucose intolerance in young adulthood (50,51).

The high frequency of congenital malformations in IDMs may be directly or indirectly associated with neuropsychological handicaps. Cerebral palsy and epilepsy are three to five times higher in IDMs compared with infants of nondiabetic mothers, but the rate of mental retardation is not different (52,53). When present, the difficulties are related to extremes of maternal age, severity of diabetes, low birth weight for gestational age, or complications during pregnancy. Psychological evaluations of children at 1, 3, and 5 yr of age suggested that, at 3 and 5 yr of age, the IDM is more vulnerable to intellectual impairment, especially if the child was born small for gestational age or if the mother's pregnancy was complicated by ketonuria (53). This has been confirmed (54). Data suggest that neurobehavioral development at birth and during childhood may be adversely affected in offspring of women with GDM whose blood glucose levels were less than optimally controlled during the pregnancy (49–51).

The question of whether the IDM has an increased likelihood of developing diabetes is important. If one parent has type 1 diabetes, it is in the range of 1–6% (55,56; see also page 7). Although family aggregates do exist, transmitted both through and within generations, a simple mode of inheritance is inconsistent with the reported data (57). Some have suggested that a polygenic multifactorial model best explains the reported observations (56). The history of maternal diabetes should not be forgotten.

REFERENCES

1. Cowett RM: The infant of the diabetic mother. In *Medical and Surgical Complications of Pregnancy: Effects on the Fetus and Newborn.* Sweet AY, Brown E, Eds. Chicago, Year Book, 1991, p. 302–19

2. Cowett RM (Ed.): Neonatal glucose metabolism. In *Principles of Perinatal-Neonatal Metabolism.* New York, Springer-Verlag, 1991, p. 356–89

3. Cowett RM: The metabolic sequelae in the infant of the diabetic mother. In *Endocrinology and Metabolism.* Cohen MP, Foa PP, Eds. *Controversies in Diabetes and Pregnancy.* Jovanovic L, sect. Ed. New York, Springer-Verlag, 1988, p. 149–71

4. Yang J, Cummings EA, O'Connell C, Jangaard K: Fetal and neonatal outcomes of diabetic pregnancies. *Obstet Gynecol* 108:644–50, 2006

5. Lee JK: Newborn resuscitation. *Pediatr Rev* 27:e52–53, 2006

6. Kinsella JP, Cutter GR, Walsh WF, Gerstmann DR, Bose CL, Hart C, Sekar KC, Auten RL, Bhutani VK, Gerdes JS, George TN, Southgate WM, Carriedo H, Couser RJ, Mammel MC, Hall DC, Pappagallo M, Sardesai S, Strain JD, Baier M, Abman SH: Early inhaled nitric oxide therapy in premature newborns with respiratory failure. *N Engl J Med* 355:354–64, 2006

7. Toker-Maimon O, Joseph LJ, Bromiker R, Schimmel MS: Neonatal cardiopulmonary arrest in the delivery room. *Pediatrics* 118:847–88, 2006

8. Cowett RM (Ed.): The infant of the diabetic mother. In *Principles of Perinatal-Neonatal Metabolism*. New York, Springer-Verlag, 1991, p. 278–98

9. Traub AI, Harley JM, Cooper TK, Maguiness S, Hadden DR: Is centralized hospital care necessary for all insulin-dependent pregnant diabetics? *Br J Obstet Gynaecol* 94:957–62, 1987

10. Hanson U, Persson B, Stangenberg M: Factors influencing neonatal morbidity in diabetic pregnancy. *Diabetes Res Clin Pract* 3:71–76, 1986

11. Wyatt JW, Frias JL, Hoyme HE, Jovanovic L, Kaaja R, Brown F, Garg S, Lee-Parritz A, Seely EW, Kerr L, Mattoo V, Tan M, and the IONS study group. Congenital anomaly rate in offspring of pre-gestational diabetic women treated with insulin lispro during pregnancy. *Diabetic Medicine* 21:2001–07, 2004

12. Rodekamp E, Harder T, Kohlhoff R, Franke K, Dudenhausen JW, Plagemann A: Long-term impact of breast-feeding on body weight and glucose tolerance in children of diabetic mothers: role of the late neonatal period and early infancy. *Diabetes Care* 28:1457–62, 2005

13. Kendrick JM, Wilson C, Elder RF, Smith CS: Reliability of reporting of self-monitoring of blood glucose in pregnant women. *J Obstet Gynecol Neonatal Nurs* 34:329–34, 2005

14. Dahlquist GG, Pundziute-Lycka A, Nystrom L, Swedish Childhood Diabetes Study Group, Diabetes Incidence Study in Sweden (DISS) Group: Birthweight and risk of type 1 diabetes in children and young adults: a population-based register study. *Diabetologia* 48:1114–47, 2005

15. ACOG Committee on Practice Bulletins: ACOG Practice Bulletin: Clinical Management Guidelines for Obstetrician-Gynecologists. Number 60, March 2005. Pregestational diabetes mellitus. *Obstet Gynecol* 105:675–85, 2005

16. Touger L, Looker HC, Krakoff J, Lindsay RS, Cook V, Knowler WC: Early growth in offspring of diabetic mothers. *Diabetes Care* 28:585–89, 2005

17. Freeman RK, Poland RL: *Guidelines for Perinatal Care*. 3rd ed. Developed by the AAP Committee on the Fetus and Newborn and the ACOG Committee on Obstetrics, Maternal and Fetal Medicine. Elk Grove, IL, American Association of Pediatrics, 1992

18. American Academy of Pediatrics: *Textbook of Neonatal Resuscitation*. Dallas, TX, American Heart Association, 1987

19. Freinkel N, Ogata E, Metzger BE: The offspring of the mother with diabetes. In *Ellenberg and Rifkin's Diabetes Mellitus: Theory and Practice*. 4th ed. Rifkin H, Porte D Jr., Eds. New York, Elsevier, 1990, p. 651

20. Kitzmiller JL, Cloherty JP, Younger MD, Tabatabaii A, Rothchild SB, Sosnko I, Epstein F, Singh S, Neff RK: Diabetic pregnancy and perinatal morbidity. *Am J Obstet Gynecol* 131:560–68, 1978

21. Metzger BE, Buchanan TA (Eds.): Diabetes and birth defects: insights from the 1980s, prevention in the 1990s. *Diabetes Spectrum* 3:149–84, 1990

22. Fuhrmann K, Reiher H, Semmler K, Fischer M, Glockner E: Prevention of congenital malformations in infants of insulin dependent diabetic mothers. *Diabetes Care* 6:219–23, 1983

23. Goldman JA, Dicker D, Feldberg D, Yeshaya A, Samuel N, Karp M: Pregnancy outcome in patients with insulin-dependent diabetes mellitus with preconceptional diabetic control: a comparative study. *Am J Obstet Gynecol* 155:193–97, 1986

24. Miller E, Hare JW, Cloherty JP, Dunn PJ, Gleason RE, Soeldner JS, Kitzmiller JL: Elevated maternal hemoglobin A1c in early pregnancy and major congenital anomalies in infants of diabetic mothers. *N Engl J Med* 304:1331–34, 1981

25. Ballard J, Holroyde J, Tsang RC, Chan G, Sutherland JM, Knowles HC: High malformation rates and decreased mortality in infants of diabetic mothers managed after the first trimester (1956–1978). *Am J Obstet Gynecol* 148:111–18, 1984

26. Way GL, Wolfe RR, Eshaghpour E, Bender RL, Jaffe RB, Ruttenberg HD: The natural history of hypertrophic cardiomyopathy in infants of diabetic mothers. *J Pediatr* 95:1020–25, 1979

27. Reeler MD, Kaplan S: Hypertrophic cardiomyopathy in infants of diabetic mothers: an update. *Am J Perinatol* 4:353–58, 1988

28. Mace S, Hirschfeld SS, Riggs T, Fanaroff AA, Merkatz IR: Echocardiographic abnormalities in infants of diabetic mothers. *J Pediatr* 95:1013–19, 1979

29. Breitweser JA, Mayer RA, Sperling MA, Psang RC, Kaplan S: Cardiac septal hypertrophy in hyperinsulinemic infants. *J Pediatr* 96:535–39, 1980

30. Halliday HL: Hypertrophic cardiomyopathy in infants of poorly controlled diabetic mothers. *Arch Dis Child* 56:258–63, 1981

31. Robert MD, Neff RK, Hubbell JP, Taeusch HW, Avery ME: Association between maternal diabetes and the respiratory distress syndrome in the newborn. *N Engl J Med* 294:357–60, 1976

32. Srinivasan G, Pildes RS, Cattamanchi G, Vooru S, Lilien LD: Plasma glucose values in normal neonates: a new look. *J Pediatr* 109:114–17, 1986

33. Lin HC, Maguire CA, Oh W, Cowett RM: Accuracy and reliability of glu-

cose reflectance meters in the high risk neonate. *J Pediatr* 115:998–1000, 1989

34. Cowett RM: Decreased response to catecholamines in the newborn: effect on glucose kinetics in the lamb. *Metabolism* 37:736–40, 1988

35. Cowett RM: Alpha adrenergic agonists stimulate neonatal glucose production less than beta adrenergic agonists in the lamb. *Metabolism* 37:831–36, 1988

36. Conrad PD, Sparks JW, Osberg I, Abrams L, Hay WW Jr: Clinical application of a new glucose analyzer in the neonatal intensive care unit: comparison with other methods. *J Pediatr* 114:281–87, 1989

37. Cowett RM, D'Amico LB: Accuracy and reliability of glucose reflectance meters in the high-risk neonate. *J Pediatr* 120:1002, 1992

38. Lilien LD, Pidles RS, Sainivasan G, Voora S, Yeh TF: Treatment of neonatal hypoglycemia with minibolus and intravenous glucose infusion. *J Pediatr* 97:295–98, 1980

39. Persson B, Gentz J, Lunell NO: Diabetes in pregnancy. In *Reviews in Perinatal Medicine. Vol. 2.* Scarpelli EM, Cosmi EV, Eds. New York, Raven, 1978, p. 1–53

40. Tsang RC, Brown DR, Steinchen JJ: Diabetes and calcium disturbances in infants of diabetic mothers. In *The Diabetic Pregnancy: A Perinatal Perspective.* Merkatz IR, Adam PAJ, Eds. New York, Grune & Stratton, 1979, p. 207–25

41. Noguchi A, Erin M, Tsang RC: Parathyroid hormone in hypocalcemia and normocalcemic infants of diabetic mothers. *J Pediatr* 97:112–14, 1980

42. Taylor PM, Wolfson J, Bright NH, Britchard EL, Derinoz MN, Watson DW: Hyperbilirubinemia in infants of diabetic mothers. *Biol Neonate* 5:289–98, 1963

43. Peevy KJ, Landaw SA, Gross SA: Hyperbilirubinemia in infants of diabetic mothers. *Pediatrics* 66:417–19, 1980

44. Stevenson DK, Ostrander CR, Cohen RS, Johnson JD, Schwartz HC: Pulmonary excretion of carbon monoxide in the human infant as an index of bilirubin production. *Eur J Pediatr* 137:255–59, 1981

45. Stevenson DK, Ostrander CR, Hopper AO, Cohen RS, Johnson JD: Pulmonary excretion of carbon monoxide as an index of bilirubin production. IIa. Evidence for possible delayed clearance of bilirubin in infants of diabetic mothers. *J Pediatr* 98:822–24, 1981

46. Farquhar JW: Prognosis for babies born to diabetic mothers in Edinburgh. *Arch Dis Child* 44:36–47, 1960

47. Bibergeil H, Bodel E, Amendt P: Diabetes and pregnancy: early and late prognoses of children of diabetic mothers. In *Early Diabetes in Early Life.* Carmerini-Davalos RA, Cole HS, Eds. New York, Academic, 1975, p. 427–34

48. Vohr BR, Lipsitt LP, Oh W: Somatic growth of children of diabetic mothers with reference to birth size. *J Pediatr* 97:196–119, 1980

49. Gerlini G, Arachi S, Gori MG, Gloria F, Bonci E, Pachi A, Zuccarini O, Fiore R, Fallucca F: Developmental aspects of the offspring of diabetic mothers. *Acta Endocrinol Suppl* 277:150–55, 1986

50. Pettitt DJ, Bennett PH, Saad MF, Charles MA, Nelson RG, Knowler WC: Abnormal glucose tolerance during pregnancy in Pima Indian women: long-term effects on offspring. *Diabetes* 40 (Suppl. 2):126–30, 1991

51. Silverman BL, Rizzo T, Green OC, Cho NH, Winter RJ, Ogata ES, Richards GE, Metzger BE: Long-term prospective evaluation of offspring of diabetic mothers. *Diabetes* 40 (Suppl. 2):121–25, 1991

52. Yssing M: Long-term prognosis of children born to mothers diabetic when pregnant. In *Early Diabetes in Early Life*. Camerini-Davalos RM, Cole HS, Eds. New York, Academic, 1975, p. 575–86

53. Stehbens JA, Baker GL, Kitchell M: Outcome at ages 1, 3, and 5 years of children born to diabetic women. *Am J Obstet Gynecol* 127:408–13, 1977

54. Rizzo T, Metzger BE, Nurns WJ, Burns K: Correlations between antepartum maternal metabolism and intelligence of offspring. *N Engl J Med* 325:911–16, 1991

55. Kobberling J, Tillil H: Risk to family members of becoming diabetic: a study on the genetics of type 1 diabetes. *Pediatr Adolesc Endocrinol* 15:26–38, 1986

56. Anderson CE, Rotter JI, Rimoin DL: Genetics of diabetes mellitus. In *Diabetes Mellitus. Vol. 5*. Rifkin H, Raskin P, Eds. Bowie, MD, Brady, 1981, p. 79

57. Simpson J: Genetics of diabetes mellitus and anomalies in offspring of diabetic mothers. In *The Diabetic Pregnancy: A Perinatal Perspective*. Merkatz IR, Adam PAJ, Eds. New York, Grune & Stratton, 1970, p. 249–60

Postpartum Follow-Up of Women with Gestational Diabetes

Highlights
Postpartum Follow-Up of
Women with Gestational Diabetes

■ Women who have had gestational diabetes have a three- to fourfold increased risk of developing type 2 diabetes in the subsequent 5–15 yr compared with the general population.

■ Postpartum, women should monitor their blood glucose levels for 1 wk; any elevation above normal should be reported to the physician.

■ At the first postpartum checkup 6–8 wk after delivery, the woman with previous GDM should undergo a 2-h 75-g oral glucose tolerance test for diabetes screening.

■ Women with previous gestational diabetes should have yearly laboratory plasma glucose measurements.

Postpartum Follow-Up of Women with Gestational Diabetes

In women with gestational diabetes mellitus (GDM), the risk of developing GDM in subsequent pregnancies and/or type 2 diabetes in the future is significantly increased compared with the general population. Women with previous GDM have a 66% risk of developing GDM in future pregnancies (1). Additionally, their risk of developing overt type 2 diabetes in the 5–15 yr subsequent to a pregnancy complicated by GDM ranges from 40 to 60%, compared with an overall 15% risk in the general population (2).

As many as 20% of women with GDM tested in the early postpartum period at 6–8 wk had an abnormal oral glucose tolerance test (OGTT) (3,4). In particular, maternal obesity, an elevated fasting glucose level during the 3-h OGTT during pregnancy, and early gestational age at the time of diagnosis of GDM (<24 wk) are significant predictors of impaired glucose tolerance or overt diabetes in the postpartum period (5). In one study, as many as 95% of women with fasting glucose concentrations in pregnancy ≥130 mg/dl (≥7.2 mmol/l) remained glucose intolerant when tested during the first year postpartum. In the same study, 67% of women whose fasting glucose levels ranged between 105 mg/dl (5.8 mmol/l) and 129 mg/dl (7.2 mmol/l) had abnormal glucose tolerance tests in the first year postpartum. Abnormal glucose tolerance during pregnancy also has long-term effects on the offspring (see page 6). For these reasons, it is important to closely monitor these women and their offspring in the months and years after pregnancy.

POSTPARTUM TESTING AND FOLLOW-UP

Immediately postpartum, the woman with previous GDM should self-monitor or have hospital staff monitor her blood glucose levels occasionally until discharged to ensure that levels have returned to normal. Random blood glucose levels in the nonpregnant state should be <10 mg/dl (<5.5 mmol/l) in the fasting state and <140 mg/dl (<7.8 mmol/l) 2 h postprandially (5). In some cases, glucose levels may remain somewhat elevated during the first 24–48 h postpartum before returning to normal levels. Once glucose levels normalize, the woman with previous GDM, to minimize the likelihood that she will become diabetic, should try to maintain a diabetes-appropriate diet. She should be advised to check her blood glucose levels on several occasions after hospital discharge, perhaps after a heavy meal. If blood glucose levels are elevated, she should notify her physician.

If a woman developed GDM very early in gestation and/or displayed a very labile blood glucose pattern, raising the suspicion that she has underlying type 1 or type 2 diabetes, the physician should ask the woman to monitor blood glucose levels closely postpartum, conveying to her concern regarding persisting diabetes. If she manifests random elevated blood glucose levels of ~200 mg/dl, a glucose tolerance test does not need to be ordered, but the women should be diagnosed as having diabetes and urgent treatment should be given. At the first postpartum checkup at 6–8 wk after delivery, all women with previous GDM should undergo a 2-h 75-g OGGT in accordance with the recommendations of the American Diabetes Association and the Fifth International Workshop-Conference on Gestational Diabetes Mellitus (6). They can then be reclassified according to their test results (7). Women with abnormal OGTT values postpartum are classified into two categories:

■ Type 2 diabetes
■ Impaired glucose tolerance (IGT)

A woman found to have type 2 diabetes should be referred for appropriate diabetes education, treatment, and follow-up. If she plans to have more children, this is an opportune time to counsel her regarding the major risks of pregnancy for women with preexisting diabetes (see page 6). She should be strongly encouraged to seek prepregnancy counseling before undertaking subsequent pregnancies. Contraceptive advice should also be given at this time, with emphasis on careful planning of future pregnancies (see page 28).

A woman with IGT should be advised of her increased risk of developing diabetes in the near future. She should be educated regarding the symptoms of overt diabetes as well as the morbidity and mortality of the chronic complications of overt diabetes. In fact, IGT alone has been associated with an increased risk for coronary artery disease. The woman with IGT should also be educated regarding various medications that adversely affect glucose metabolism, including some oral contraceptives, thiazide diuretics, steroids, and β-blockers. If obese, the woman should be urged to reduce her body weight by 5–7%. Depending on the degree of severity of glucose intolerance, she should be advised to have interval blood glucose levels to ensure early detection of overt diabetes, especially if future pregnancies are anticipated.

A woman with a normal postpartum OGTT should likewise be counseled regarding her risk of developing GDM in future pregnancies and her risk of developing type 2 diabetes as outlined above. Older obese women especially are at increased risk to develop recurrent GDM (8). If obese, a woman should be strongly encouraged to lose weight in that obesity is not only a significant risk factor for GDM in subsequent pregnancies but is also predictive of type 2 diabetes in future years. Obese women have a 50–75% risk of developing type 2 diabetes, whereas women with previous GDM of ideal body weight have a 25% risk of developing type 2 diabetes (2,5,9). This is an opportune time to emphasize these risks and advise her of her opportunity to perhaps reduce them and delay the onset of overt diabetes with its attendant morbidity and mortality. The physician should encourage the woman to see a dietitian, who can assist her in developing a plan for safe effective weight loss. Encouraging the woman to also develop an exercise program appropriate for her is advisable.

YEARLY FOLLOW-UP AND COUNSELING

Long-term follow-up of women with previous GDM is vital and must be individualized. Every woman, at the minimum, should have a yearly fasting plasma glucose measurement. Levels >100 mg/dl (>5.6 mmol/l) deserve medical intervention or diet/exercise counseling. At this yearly follow-up, the physician can not only assess the woman's glucose level, but also evaluate her efforts at weight reduction and her plans for a future pregnancy. During these visits, the physician should also inquire about the woman's offspring, especially with regard to body weight and glucose intolerance. As noted on page 150, infants of diabetic mothers have an increased risk of obesity in adolescence and may also have an increased risk of developing glucose intolerance in young adulthood. These follow-up visits provide an excellent opportunity to review for the woman her specific risks and those of her offspring.

REFERENCES

1. Philipson EH, Super DM: Gestational diabetes mellitus: does it recur in subsequent pregnancy? *Am J Obstet Gynecol* 160:1324–31, 1989

2. O'Sullivan JB: Diabetes mellitus after GDM. *Diabetes* 40 (Suppl. 2):131–39, 1991

3. Catalano PM, Vargo KM, Bernstein IM, Aminis B: Incidence and risk factors associated with abnormal postpartum glucose tolerance in women with gestational diabetes. *Am J Obstet Gynecol* 165:914–19, 1991

4. Kjos SL, Buchanan TA, Greenspoon JS, Montovo M, Bernstein GS, Mestman JH: Gestational diabetes mellitus: the prevalence of glucose intolerance and diabetes mellitus in the first two months postpartum. *Am J Obstet Gynecol* 163:93–98, 1990

5. Dornhorst A, Bailey PC, Anyaoku V, Elkeles RS, Johnston DB, Beard RW: Abnormalities of glucose tolerance following gestational diabetes. *Q J Med* 284:1219–28, 1990

6. Expert Committee on the Diagnosis and Classification of Diabetes Mellitus: Report of the Expert Committee on the Diagnosis and Classification of Diabetes Mellitus. *Diabetes Care* 26 (Suppl. 1):S5–20, 2002

7. Metzger BE, Coustan DR: Summary and recommendations of the Fifth International Workshop-Conference on Gestational Diabetes Mellitus. *Diabetes Care* 30 (Suppl. 2):S251–60, 2007

8. Dooley SL, Metzger BE, Cho NH: Gestational diabetes mellitus, influence of race on disease prevalence and perinatal outcome in a U.S. population. *Diabetes* 40 (Suppl. 2):25–29, 1991

9. O'Sullivan JB: Body weight and subsequent diabetes mellitus. *JAMA* 248:949–52, 1982

Index

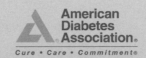
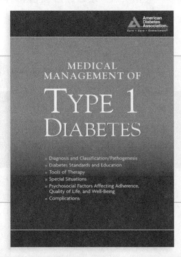
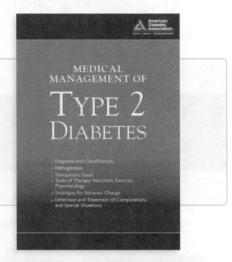
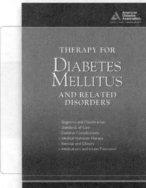
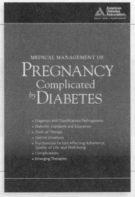
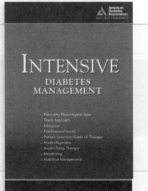